MY JOURNEY TO WELLNESS

How I Beat Cancer Naturally

Tips on Prevention

Necessary Cleanses for Optimal Health

By Ursula Kaiser

www.Ursula Kaiser.com

Published in the United States

First Edition

Book Cover Painted by Ursula Kaiser

DISCLAIMER

This book details the Author's personal experiences with and opinions about cancer. Neither the author nor the publisher is a healthcare provider.

This book is providing the Author's life journey and makes no representations or warranties of any kind with respect to this book or its contents. The Author and publisher do not represent or warrant that the information accessible via this book is accurate, complete, or current.

The statements made about products and services have not been evaluated by the US Food and Drug Administration. They are not intended to diagnose, treat, cure, or prevent any condition or disease. Please consult with your own physician or healthcare specialist regarding the suggestions and recommendations made in this book.

Except where specifically stated neither Author or Publisher nor any other contributors or other representatives will be liable for damages arising out of or in connection with the use of this book. This is a comprehensive limitation of liability that applies to all damages of any kind, including without limitation compensatory; direct, indirect, or consequential damages, loss of date, income or profit, loss of or damage to property and claims of third parties.

You must understand that this book is not intended as a substitute for consultation with a licensed healthcare practitioner, such as your physician. Before you begin any healthcare program, or change your lifestyle in any way, you will consult your physician or other licensed healthcare practitioner to insure that you are in good health and that the examples contained in this book will not harm you. This book provides the reader content related to topics concerning physical and or mental health issues. As such, use of this book implies your acceptance of this disclaimer.

TABLE OF CONTENTS

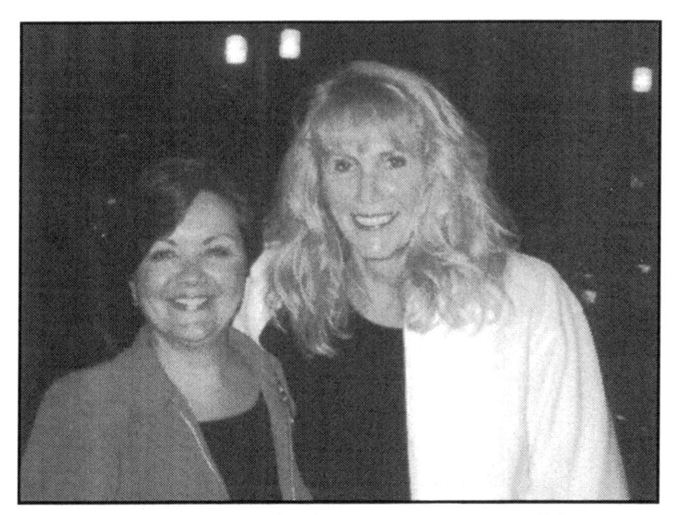

Vanda Bandera (left) & Ursula Kaiser (right)

DEDICATION

I WOULD LIKE TO DEDICATE THIS BOOK in loving memory to my best friend Vanda Bandera. I met Vanda on the phone booking my airline tickets and one day she said, "That is it Ursula; we need to meet." I expected to find this tall strong woman and when we met she was this short little dynamo and we became fast friends immediately.

Vanda was born in Italy and came to the United States at the age of 9 and did not speak English. She told me stories of how her classmates teased her about her broken English which is where she got her hard as nails disposition. Vanda was a pistol and loved to argue Italian style.

I remember her telling me stories of the long dragged out verbal fights she had with her mother and I even witnessed them firsthand in the kitchen. Wow! It amazed me how they would go at it in Italian – I would never get away with speaking to my mother that way! This family was very intense, but after the arguments would settle, they truly were the most loving and passionate people I have ever met.

I quickly became part of the family and was invited to all of their family functions. Vanda would call me and say, "Hey Ursula, next Saturday you have to be at this church (Catholic) in Chicago for some special holiday or mass." She would say "Ursula I am not asking, I am telling you to be there!" Of course I would show up and on time ...

One thing about Vanda that would drive me crazy was she was never on time. That girl would keep me waiting for hours. I used to get so frustrated and found it so disrespectful. Instead of acting out German style (angry), I quickly learned to plan around her crazy schedule so it would not ruin our relationship because she was such a beautiful soul and full of life.

However, 6 months before Vanda passed away, I was diagnosed with cancer too! How is this possible? How am I going to look her in the face and tell her what I was just told by the doctors? I had been watching my friend fight

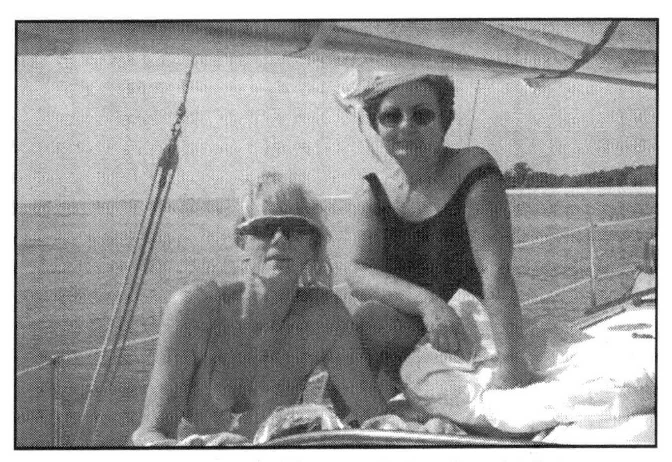

Ursula Kaiser (left) & Vanda Bandera (right)

for her life and now we had to do it together, literally. I was diagnosed and given 3 – 6 months to live. That day came and all we could do is cry in each other arms and wonder why us! Two dynamic, lively, spirited women having to fight for our lives just did not seem fair. After watching Vanda go through her chemo and radiation, I knew that I would not go down that path as you will find in my story.

So this book is dedicated to Vanda for cheerleading me on from above. I miss you, Dear Friend, and know you are smiling from above as I finally finish my book and share it with others who are fighting their own battle or who continue to seek health and wellness naturally.

FORWARD

While floating totally relaxed and meditating in the mineral pool at the Ritz Carlton, a voice interrupts my trance. I am startled out of my relaxed state back to reality with a concerned voice asking me, "Are you alright? Are you okay?" This person, Leslie, thought I had drowned and died in the pool. We talk for a few moments and I hear sadness in her voice. Leslie shares that she is fighting breast cancer and has just finished the last round of chemotherapy, and had fears of dying. I say, "I had cancer 6 years ago and the doctors gave me 3 - 6 months to live." I then begin to tell her my story...

For five years I have been talking about writing this book and lecturing about alternative healing. Due to a lawsuit I was involved in with a multi-million dollar company, my lawyer advised me not to write this book. He told me, "The jury will think you are totally whacked out." The lawsuit had to do with a successful kitchen utensils company that I started in 1974, way before my cancer.

First lesson in the healing process – **Learn How to Let Go!** You have to learn how to detach from all stressful situations and not let your body suffer. I then realized how STRESS is very damaging to every aspect of a person's mental, emotional, physical and spiritual life. You can eat all the right foods and do all the right things, but your emotions can still make your body's system quite acidic. I cannot tell you how VERY important it is to work on your emotions.

So, back to the beginning. I listened to my attorney and did not write my book. I waited until this moment in time. It is now time to speak my truth which is my passion in life, or my mission as you might say, to help others fighting their own battles with cancer. I have dreamt of telling my story to others that are filled with fear when they are given a death sentence!

So, my dear friend, this book is for you. Know that you can beat any disease in your life, especially CANCER. However, it will take your will to live, the determination to make all the necessary life style changes in your life, discipline to stay on track, ability to reduce all stress in your life, and you must keep a positive attitude at all times. May my journey assist you in your fight and I hope to meet you one day soon!

We are each responsible for
all of our experiences.
~ Louise L. Hay

ACKNOWLEDGEMENTS

I would like to thank the following friends that have shared their stories, journey, and healing information that added to this book. Thank you Judy Sabers for your friendship and sharing our continued journey to health and wellness, my dear cousin Dr. Rainer for being open minded and trying new ways to approach your illness, to Noel Inniss for sharing your thoughts and beliefs on consciousness which is truly important, to Joyce Pellegrini who assisted me with the completion of this book and your own story and importance of how your emotions drive the body, to Charles Marble for your vast knowledge of the body, cleanses, remedies, and awesome recipes contributed, and to Patti Acerra who assisted me in writing my story.

I also want to thank all my friends in Chicago and Naples for your support through my time of healing.

To all my friends and family in Germany that were against my going the alternative route! You know me. "My GERMAN disposition" kicked butt and I proved you wrong!

PART 1

MY JOURNEY TO WELLNESS

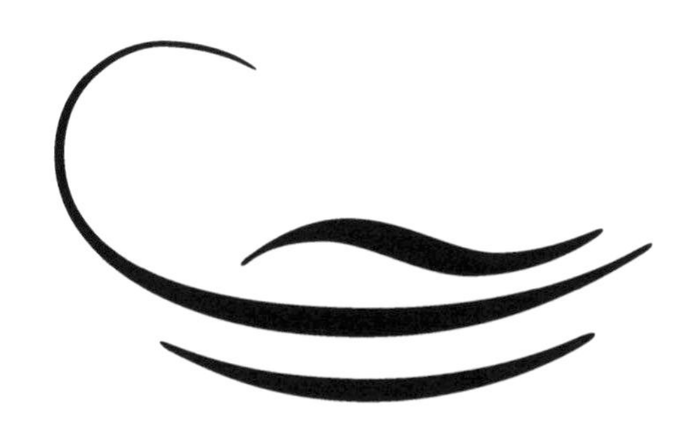

Chapter 1
Courage

LITTLE DID I KNOW WHEN I WENT TO sleep on June 9, 1999, that I was being pushed into a journey that would take mountains of courage and years of time. Courage that I didn't know I had and time that I was afraid would run out!

On that June evening almost a decade ago, I woke up to use the bathroom in the middle of the night, and was shocked to find that I was bleeding profusely from my vagina. I passed 50 - 60 large blood clots while my mind reeled with disbelief and panic. Rushing to the phone and doing my best to speak clearly, I called several good friends. Help! I'm bleeding to death! Come right now! I'm dying!

Each friend told me to wait until the next day. (Of course, it WAS the middle of the night.) "Don't worry," they said. "It is part of menopause." "You'll be fine." I managed to relax myself and returned to bed.

The next morning I drove to the clinic to meet with my gynecologist. He told me I had a cyst which was "no big deal." "Don't worry, we can schedule you for surgery tomorrow; it will take about 40 minutes." I sighed with relief. OK, so it was going to mess up my plans for a day or two. At least I wasn't dying. I made the arrangements for the following day.

When the *anesthesiologist* was putting me under, I remember making a mental list of all the things I had to do that afternoon while I was recuperating. As you will find out, I am an "A" type personality, and NO minutes go wasted.

Forty minutes of surgery dragged into four hours. When I came partially to consciousness in the recovery room, the first person I saw was my gynecologist. Still groggy from the anesthesia, I smiled as he told me not to worry about anything. What did I have to worry about? I left without really speaking to anyone. I had planned to be up and about that afternoon, packing for a trip that I had planned for the end of the week.

I slept for 24 hours. Always the healthy athlete, I was not used to taking drugs for anything. I was also a vegetarian. I prided myself on being fit and vibrant. When I got up the next day, I could hardly walk. I called Dr. Ramsey's office to speak to him. I was told that while I was in surgery to have a cyst removed, they had removed one of my ovaries.

I went through with my mini-vacation and was away from home for about six days. Lots of sunshine would help my healing. I had a follow-up appointment with Dr. Ramsey scheduled for several weeks in the future. The day after I returned home, Dr. Ramsey called me to come in to see him sooner. Like right away. Like NOW! As I stood in his office (once again with a mental list of everything else I could be doing), he told me he had removed BOTH my ovaries during the surgery for my cyst removal. No wonder I slept for so long! No wonder I couldn't walk the next day! "Your ovaries didn't look good, so I took them out while I had you under, and sent them to the pathology lab. The pathology report confirmed my suspicions. You have cancer."

What was he saying? Is he talking to me? My thoughts were tumbling all over each other. Somehow my mind registered that he wanted me back in for more surgery. Because of the cancer findings, he wanted to perform a total hysterectomy. "Oh yeah, by the way, I took out your lymph nodes too, which were positive," he said. Both ovaries and some lymph nodes and now he wants my uterus, too... Cancer ...

I was devastated; my spirit crushed. Everything was moving so fast. What happened to, "It's only a cyst?" Dr. Ramsey was still speaking. "It needs to be done right away - immediately. After the surgery, you'll need radiation, of course." Of course? Radiation of course? I nodded, thanked him, and left.

At home I went on my knees and cried for a long time asking God "why me."

The next day I went to Northwestern Hospital in Chicago for a second opinion with Dr. Little. He confirmed Dr. Ramsey's opinion. "Yes, you'll need surgery. Yes, you'll need radiation immediately after." For a moment, feeling defeated and confused, I asked what the side affects of radiation were. He quickly outlined them: damaging normal healthy cells near cancer area, pain, nausea, vomiting, fatigue, anemia, lymph edema, infections, loss of hair, etc.

Nausea, vomiting, hair loss, fatigue, malaise, low blood count, cough, diarrhea, cramps, scaring, leukemia, urinary and bowel problems (wearing a bag for elimination for the rest of my life.) I asked what the chances were of having any side effects. Twenty percent was the answer. That was too high for me. I nodded, thanked him, and left.

Within the week, I was at the University of Loyola Hospital in the suburbs of Chicago. There

I received almost the same opinion. Yes, I needed surgery. Yes, I would need radiation immediately after. Then they threw something else into the pot. "You'll need chemotherapy, too." And, of course, I needed it all right away. RIGHT away. Talk about being pressured. I was going to die of fright before the cancer could kill me.

So I returned to Hinsdale Hospital and allowed Dr. Ramsey (accompanied by an oncologist) to perform the surgery. This was all within ten days of my last appointment with Dr. Ramsey. They cut me wide open from my xyphoid (lower abdominal area) to the center of my chest. They took out lymph nodes under my breast. After the surgery I needed time to heal and catch my breath. Dr. Ramsey was really pushing me to begin the radiation immediately. But I wouldn't do it. I just wanted to be left alone. As soon as I could manage, I returned to Northwestern and Loyola to get a "second" opinion (for the second time!) I didn't know whether to do radiation and chemotherapy, or just radiation or just chemotherapy, or NOTHING. I went to ask for more information to make a decision. Armed with all my pathology reports from my first AND second surgery, I asked various doctors at both hospitals to help me understand. They had taken out my ovaries during my first surgery. They had taken out my uterus and lymph nodes during the second surgery. Where was the cancer? Was there any left? What could they tell me?

The hospitals did not agree. Loyola said after the 2nd surgery that I had uterine AND ovarian cancer. Northwestern told me that I had ovarian cancer which spread to the lymph nodes. They both confirmed their original recommendations. Northwestern said radiation was the course of action, and Loyola urged for both radiation and chemotherapy.

Feeling totally drained, confused, and powerless, I agreed to the treatments. I began to "make a bed" for my radiation. This is a process which you are fitted for the machine so that you do not move during treatment. Every time I went to get sized up for my hips, I would be filled with dread lying under that huge machine. I was so uncomfortable with the whole environment, too. During my third and last fitting, lying there staring up at that monster of a machine, I heard someone or something telling me to **"get up and go".** So that's exactly what I did. I left and never went back. I cancelled all radiation appointments with Loyola and Northwestern Hospitals. I didn't want anything to do with it. I didn't want the side effects. Somehow, this simple act helped me to regain my power back.

The doctor at Northwestern in charge of the radiation department actually called me at home and aggressively told me that if I didn't come in to get the radiation, I was giving myself a death sentence with fewer than three months to live. It amazed me that he was saying this to me over the phone! He was young, brash, and very confident that I would die very soon. But I didn't believe it. When I didn't respond, the certified letters started coming. They were confirming that I left treatment of my own free will on my own decision. They warned me that I was being irresponsible and outlined the consequences (death). I felt angry and confused. But I still wouldn't go back.

Dr. Ramsey went on his knees pleading (I was like a sister) and begged that if I wouldn't do radiation at least do Tomoxifen. I bought the Tomoxifen and looked at the side effects listed on the package. I took it for one week. In one week I gained ten pounds, my emotions were up and down like a roller coaster, (which is VERY unusual for a German), and I felt depressed. I decided to quit the drug after just one week.

Every thought we think is
creating our future.
~ Louise L. Hay

Chapter 2
Who Am I?

I THINK IT'S IMPORTANT TO TELL YOU A little bit about me. We all make decisions based on our past, and I am no exception.

I was raised in a small town in Germany called Rendsburg. Our biggest attraction is the Kaiser Wilhelm canal that connects the Baltic Sea with the Mighty North Sea. As a young girl, I would watch all the ocean liners and freight ships from different countries passing by. They all seemed so mysterious to me and it touched my life. I spent hours and hours studying all the flags from the world that were passing me by. I would find the countries on the globe and read whatever I could find about them. I would sit at the canal, dreaming that one day I would travel to all the continents. I spent many, many days and hours at that canal, watching the people on the ships. Sometimes they would wave to me and call out in different languages: French, Russian, Chinese...

The other attraction in town was the hanging ferry, which connected the towns across the canal. This ferry was free, and my friends and I would travel back and forth on it all day until the guard got tired of us. For young children it was fascinating and time just flew by. I was always late for supper and many times my brother was sent to find me and bring me home. I was always in trouble for spending too much time at the canal.

On weekends the whole family would walk on the canal (it looked like a boardwalk). We would always end up, as the other families did, at our favorite café for ice cream.

I told my parents at the age of 12 that I intended to move far away from Germany and kept telling them that until I was 21. My urge to see the world increased as I grew older. I studied business in Germany with a girlfriend. We were the first females in the class. It was a time when females were rarely hired in upper management.

"Ursula, it seems you were born to break every rule," my father would say. They called me the black sheep. Even the school system made me restless. I couldn't connect with the teachers and they couldn't connect with me. I did not act like a proper German girl. Honestly, I didn't FEEL like a "proper German girl." I couldn't connect with my mother, either. She would say, "Ursula, you are never homesick: you are always *fernweh* sick (which means far-away sick). I wanted to be anywhere else but where I was born.

Ever since I was young, I knew I had to explore who I was. Family and friends used to say "this is it." Meaning, you get what you see. All emotional issues were swept under the rug. Don't stir anything up. I knew I needed to explore myself. I wasn't happy this way. There had to be more in life and I wanted it.

When I turned 19, I began making my plans to go to South Africa, America, or Australia. It was very difficult to get a working permit for South Africa. By the time I was 21 I had decided to take off, instead, for New York and Broadway. The only working permit for the United States was as an au pair for a family. This was not the glamour I had in mind, but I accepted the offer just to get out of Germany. Remember, I was young and restless. I had just turned 21 and was full of confidence. With $5 in my pocket, I landed in New York, not knowing anyone, not even the family who would be picking me up.

I worked 70 hours per week for the family that was sponsoring me. I had to serve their daughters, who actually rang a bell when they wanted my service. This was not my idea of independence. Within 6 months of working there and saving all my money, I told them I was leaving. I paid them back for my flight and had $60 left. From there I went to Chicago with a friend I had made - another German girl. She had relatives in Chicago so we hopped on the first bus out of New York.

My first job in Chicago was as a bookkeeper. Soon I found another part-time job in a German delicatessen on Lincoln Avenue. At night I started at Heidelberger Fass Restaurant as my third job. I kept a record of all the money I was making and saved $10,000 my first year. That was a lot of money in German marks. I went home on vacation to visit my parents, my girlfriends and practically spent it all.

I came back to America ready to work and make more money when I realized that I was not the type who could work for anyone else. I studied to get my own import license. The owner of a small import company, Mr. Kalkus, asked me if I could help him out and run the company. The gentleman was older and mostly on the road selling and delivering, so it was fun to work by myself. I put my business education to good use. My first tradeshow was at Navy Pier. I rented

During the next 15 years, I fulfilled all of my dreams of travelling professionally and personally all over the world, skied often, biked all over the United States, worked hard and played hard "Life was great"!

Dying of Cancer was never on the agenda...

Self-approval and
self-acceptance in the now
are the keys to positive change.
~ Louise L. Hay

Chapter 3
Now What?

SO NOW WHAT? NOW THAT I REFUSED chemotherapy, refused radiation, refused Tomaxofen which is a cancer drug, what am I going to do?

I picked up a few books on cancer and began to read. I needed more information. I needed to see if there was another way to win against this disease called cancer! I needed **HOPE...**

I read several books like Cancer Battle, Cancer is Not a Disease, Fighting Cancer with Nutrition, to name a few. These were my first steps toward taking total responsibility for my health. This was the true beginning of my journey into the world of healing. All my friends and all of the doctors had their opinions of what I should do.

My friends that believed in alternative healing said **"Good for you... go find your path."** One said "I can heal you; come visit me" but I didn't want to put myself in one person's hands. I wanted to make my decisions based on knowledge and instinct - not fear or desperation.

One alternative health friend told me about a clinic in Mexico. The clinic had been recommended by another doctor in New Mexico. It was called Regenesis. I flew there with my friend Vanda who was suffering with breast cancer that had spread. When we arrived at this clinic, we were astounded. It was a filthy small place. We made jokes about our disappointments. "What, no wine? No TV? No gourmet food?" We thought the food was absolutely awful, even though it was organic and vegetarian.

I liked that the director of Regenesis he was both a doctor and scientist, trained in Germany / Europe, but from South Africa. I respected him and felt confident in his knowledge. This was the first time I was exposed to colonics. It was fewer than six weeks after my second surgery and my whole body hurt. They began giving us coffee enemas. "Oh my God," I thought. "What am I doing here?"

It was at this clinic that we met a young lady from Milwaukee who also had breast cancer. Vanda made instant friends with her. She was to play a very important part in another part of our journey. More details will come on this later.

One night the Director of the clinic sat Vanda and I down and tore us apart. "Who do you think you are asking for wine and TV and special food?" He was angry! "You are making much too light of the fact that you NEED to be here. This is not a vacation. This is serious. If you don't turn around in a very short period of time, you will be expelled from the clinic." He now had our attention.

We gave ourselves a serious attitude adjustment and became much more committed to our health. It was the first time I heard anyone say that it was up to me to stop the cancer in my body. No fruit, no sugar, no starches, no yeast. And the director said, "Ursula, you're German. You are strong; if you pull yourself together, you can do it." Then he pointed at my happy, fun loving Italian friend Vanda and said to her "You, especially, have to shape up!"

That day it really sunk in that I wasn't just going to a health clinic for a week or a month to cure my cancer. I would need to take the regime that I was learning and keep it up for a year to make sure that all the cancer in my body was gone. That meant I would have to write down everything they were telling me to do so that I would do it on my own. I was in school to learn how to live and rid my body of this toxic disease.

We left the clinic after 4 days. Vanda became friends with the Milwaukee girl and kept in touch; we found out that she had gone to another clinic in Mexico. Vanda tried to call her there, dialed the wrong number, and mistakenly got in touch with another woman named Judy from South Dakota who told us about yet ANOTHER clinic in Mexico. To this day, I do not believe it was a "mistaken wrong number." Judy and I are still friends today.

I had been researching clinics in the United States because I did not want to go back to Mexico. But Vanda insisted, and because of our friendship, I went along. We went for a little over two weeks of detoxification. We did IVs of vitamins every day for four hours. We also did coffee enemas every day. The theory was to alkalize the body and stimulate the organs. We had fun together and made a party out of it. There was a pool there and tennis court. The "clinic" was a very nice huge house that had been turned into a health center, but at night the girl from Milwaukee used to scream, and they wouldn't give her the pain shots she was supposed to have. I stayed with her at night to comfort her. We continued to stay at that clinic even though I was very skeptical of the care. The nurses didn't speak English and it was not a very professional atmosphere. Something just didn't seem right. Then one morning a couple that came there for detoxing explained to us that the REAL clinic was in Tijuana and that the clinic we were at was just an offshoot of the bigger clinic. Vanda and I immediately told the directors that we wanted to go and we are going to make arrangements to leave, but they locked us in! During the early morning light, we quietly left and went to the clinic in Tijuana. By this time I was getting frustrated with Vanda, and we had a fight.

When we got to the clinic in Tijuana, things seemed to be better. The nurses were very good, spoke English, and seemed very professional. They performed a Live Blood Cell Analysis on us - something I had never had done before. It was the first time I had looked at my blood and seen my own cells. They were all sticking together and my white cells were not moving at all. It was not a pretty picture. "Is that normal?" I asked. "No," they said. "You're in pretty bad shape." I had a horrible ring around my cells. Everything was very unhealthy looking and it depressed me. The operation had only taken care of some of the cancer. I needed to get the rest of the cancer out of my system.

We stayed there for two weeks. I ate apricot pits (which contain B17 also known as laetrile, a known cancer killer) every day and started all over with the coffee enemas. We had breath workshops. Putting oxygen in the body helps stop the cancer. At first I couldn't even breathe and hold my breath for very long because of the surgeries. The camaraderie felt good. We were a team - we knew we needed to be strict and we were in it together. We all supported and inspired each other while adding humor to lift our spirits as well as our spirituality. At times, the husbands even came to the clinic to visit.

The theory here was the same as at Regenesis - starve the Cancer. Do that by eliminating starches, sugar, etc. We had to be strict. Potatoes, rice, bread, pasta, could no longer be part of our diet. How long you have to do this depends on what state you're in. Sometimes it's only for three to six months. Sometimes it's for much longer.

Just a note on something very radically wrong here. In the radiation rooms of large hospitals, COOKIES are made available after radiation. Cookies are loaded with sugar. Sugar feeds cancer. Get the picture? I'm sure these people are trying to be comforting, but instead they are being harmful.

It was about six weeks after my first visit to Mexico. I was back in Chicago. This is when I learned of a test called the AMAS test, which can measure cancer cells in your body. That test showed that I still had too many cancer cells. Suddenly I was filled with fear again. I had pain

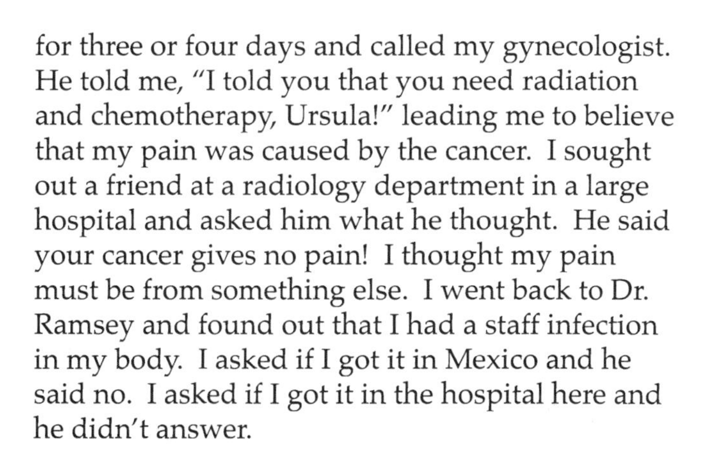

for three or four days and called my gynecologist. He told me, "I told you that you need radiation and chemotherapy, Ursula!" leading me to believe that my pain was caused by the cancer. I sought out a friend at a radiology department in a large hospital and asked him what he thought. He said your cancer gives no pain! I thought my pain must be from something else. I went back to Dr. Ramsey and found out that I had a staff infection in my body. I asked if I got it in Mexico and he said no. I asked if I got it in the hospital here and he didn't answer.

I read more books, did more research, found out more information. Information about remedies as simple as teas brewed specifically to fight cancer to intricate frequency machines that do the same thing. There was so much information available to me!

A friend in New Orleans had been diagnosed with breast cancer and given three months to live. She told me about a doctor in St. Augustine who worked with a frequency machine that helped. (Frequency will be explained in another chapter.) I went to St. Augustine and had frequency treatments for three days (4 hours a day.) I had to fly to Naples and then drive to Orlando crying the whole way. After the first day, I asked if I could do all the treatments in one day and get it over with. I guess my "type A" personality was till the death. But alternative health is not a quick fix. It's not like having surgery. It takes time and dedication. I sat in the office for 3 days while the doctor worked on layers and layers of infection in my body by touching the tip of my thumbnail and index finger with probes hooked up to the frequency machine. The machine showed what was excessive or deficient throughout my body. It was Thanksgiving weekend. I spent most of the time driving back and forth from St. Augustine to Naples CRYING...

I want to stress here that my emotions were running wild. I had a successful business in Chicago that needed my attention. I was in the midst of a lawsuit. I had lost my best customer and was worried about finances... and I had just built my dream home in Vail, Colorado. One of my employees had died of cancer, and one was seriously ill with cancer and leukemia in advanced stages and had to stay home. I had to do both their jobs on my own because I had no money to hire anyone else. I barely left the warehouse. I napped, worked, and cleansed over and over again and healed myself at the same time.

If you had asked me back then, "What would you do if I had cancer?" I would have said "I'd go to the Himalayas and meditate for six months until I keeled over." That's how I always thought I would handle a death sentence. Now here I was working my butt off at the warehouse all day. Working a full eight hours and napping and cleansing and napping and cleansing. I was there from 7 a.m. to 11 p.m. I was fighting cancer. I was fighting for my business, to stay awake, and alive. My dear friends took shifts and came to assist me through this time in my life. I am so very grateful for their loving friendship and support. Even an old boyfriend came in to help me, side by side with my current boyfriend. I learned how to accept help. I learned that I could not control everything. Little by little, this journey for my health taught me a lot about things I would never have thought of before.

During this time my brother, Gerhard, wanted to come and help me at the warehouse. He was going to come from Germany and help me. I declined because he was very allopathic oriented and I didn't want anyone around me to be negative about what I was doing. He was very supportive of me and wanted to help anyway, so I told him to give me some money to help pay for my healing in Mexico. "If it doesn't work and I die, you'll get all of the money that we're going to inherit from Mom's house." I said, "so you might as well dish some out now." He did, and I paid him every penny back after my healing!

I had Plan A, Plan B, Plan C, and Plan D all lined up to help get new clients to make up the slack from losing my best customer. I was stressed and worried about money and my business. However, by some miracle I landed the

Martha Stewart account which saved my business and made it profitable once again. It was now time to sell it and concentrate on my healing. It is very important to relieve all the stress you have, however you can, when you are trying to heal.

I was taking the "Gonzalez Supplement Program" which consisted of $2,000 worth of vitamins a month. The tea I was taking was $500 per month. I spent about $4,000 a month on healing for six months straight. Now that I've been through this ordeal I know that you can fight cancer and it will not be that costly for you. **Ignorance is expensive**. **Ignorance about good health is deadly.**

I had a friend who was an "alternative oncologist." He came and gave Vanda and I IVs of vitamins. He said cancer was like a crossword puzzle. He told me I couldn't do enough for my body in the state I was in. He told me to do everything I could and the body would heal itself of the cancer. Unfortunately, he went back to being a traditional oncologist because he couldn't support his family being an alternative doctor.

During this battle I had to keep my business going until I could sell it, and to keep my LIFE going until I could heal it. I got a call from my friend Vanda. She said, "You need to go to Honduras for me tomorrow." "What?" "Are you crazy?" "Tomorrow?" I had a closing on my house in Vail that week. There was no way I could go to Honduras.

But Vanda was persistent. President Reagan had passed legislation that would allow US citizens to travel to different countries and return with a six month supply of any drug that you needed for your cancer treatment. (President Reagan had cancer). Vanda had heard of a "miracle drug" that could only be found in Honduras. She was too weak to go herself. It was up to me.

"I don't care about your closing," said my mild-mannered Italian friend. "This is life and death. If you don't go, I'll die."

So the next day, I found myself on a plane, headed for Honduras. There was no way I could have lived with myself had I not done this for Vanda. When I landed in a very small airport, there was no one there who spoke English. I only knew where to go because there was a woman standing in the terminal with a handwritten sign in her hand with my name on it. I accompanied her into the car and we proceeded to drive and drive. Over 45 minutes of driving, deep into the mountains. By now I wasn't the least bit worried about my cancer. I had $12,000 in my pocket and everyone must have known it, because those were the arrangements that had been made. The only thing I was worried about was being robbed and killed and left along the roadside.

Finally, we arrived at a house in the mountains. The men there produced a drug and a syringe and were gesturing for me to inject myself right then and there. They said that before I left with the drug, they had to be sure that I could inject it properly into my body. I tried to explain that the drug was not for me, but for Vanda.

When I finally made them understand, they told me that they didn't care WHO it was for. Unless I learned how to inject it properly, I was not leaving with the drug. To my astonishment, they roughly jabbed a very long needle into the front of my left thigh. WHAM. Then they gave me a room to rest in. The next day they informed me that they wanted to watch me inject the drug. I was to do it in the other thigh. After several hesitant moments I thrust the needle into my thigh just barely indenting my skin. Obviously, I didn't have the technique right. After a few more feeble attempts, they took the needle from me and WHAM... jabbed my right thigh and walked out of the room.

The next day when they gestured for me to inject the drug, I did it right because I wanted to get the hell out of there. I could hardly move but off I went back to the United States to deliver the drug to Vanda. Unfortunately, the drug never helped her. She was already in too bad of shape. Just over two months later, she fell into a coma and died in the hospital. She admitted before she died that she never had stuck to her program of juicing, and had not done her detoxing like she was supposed to. She still had the "mindset" of a miracle drug. But at least I had done what she asked me to do.

I lovingly forgive and release all the past. I choose to fill my world with joy. I love and approve of myself.

~ Louise L. Hay

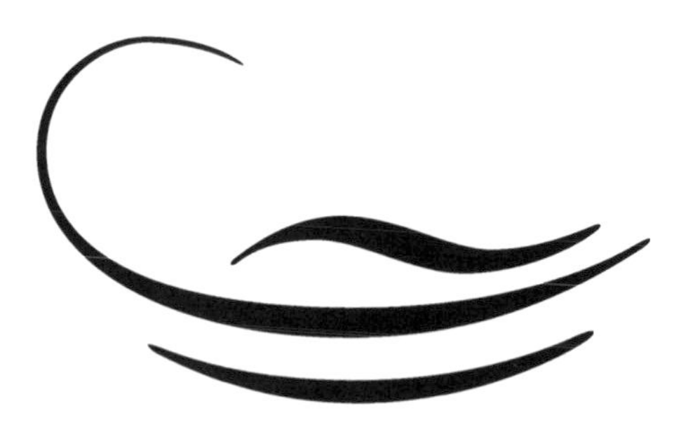

Chapter 4

One And A Half Years Later...

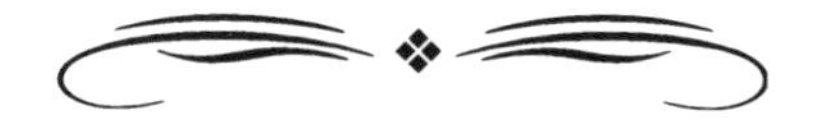

ONE AND A HALF YEARS LATER, I STILL had pain in my right lower abdomen. Whenever I went to Dr. Ramsey, he would say, "I know Ursula. You still need radiation; we're not done yet." My friend Judy found an alternative cancer clinic in Tulsa, Oklahoma. Judy and I got "recruited" to go to the clinic because of our conditions. The clinic would pay for our flights there and back and for the vitamins, and all we needed to do was give the clinic our insurance cards.

They had a PET scanner that showed how much cancer was in our bodies. We took our pathology reports with us, as per their instructions. They gave us a physical and organized us for the PET scan. They also set up appointments for us to see the resident doctor. The doctor was just one floor up from where we were having our PET scan taken... and yet... (we found out later) the doctor had no idea that when you were in the PET scan, you couldn't move for three hours. He also had no idea that we were scheduled for the PET scan at the same time and wondered why I hadn't kept my appointment. This made me feel uncomfortable. Like the right hand not knowing what the left hand was doing. Nobody was seeing the whole picture. When the technician finished with the PET scan, I asked him what the results were. He told me that he could read it but was not allowed to tell me anything because he told a patient one time and almost got sued and kicked out of the hospital. He was only allowed to tell his findings to the doctor. The doctor would have to tell me.

But when I finally made it to my appointment (with the doctor upstairs), he didn't even know what the PET scan was and didn't know how to read it. This occurred directly upstairs in the same facility. The third doctor I saw in this same facility merely told me the same thing I'd been hearing all along, that I needed to come back for 6 weeks and have "light" chemo. I needed a very light dosage of chemotherapy over a longer period of time so I wouldn't lose my hair.

This didn't sound like such an "alternative" to me. Judy and I were receiving drip vitamins in this facility and struck up a conversation with the man sitting next to us. We had seen him before in the clinic and wanted to know how he was doing. We asked him which vitamin he was "dripping" and he answered that he was dripping on chemotherapy! Meanwhile, he was drinking a Diet Coke! This was supposed to be an alternative health clinic and they were letting him drink a diet Coke while sitting and receiving chemotherapy drips. Unbelievable! This man told us much later that he thought he was still alive only because he continued, on his own, to drink Essiac Tea the whole time he was on chemotherapy.

This clinic in Tulsa gave us vitamins to take home and classes on nutrition and food. However, they really tried to convince us to come back for light chemo. They did that with everybody.

Every year I do a detoxification program and totally cleanse my body internally. This is how I've stayed clean of cancer for almost ten years now. It's how I intend to stay clean of cancer for the rest of my life. I also take the "AMAS" test every year from Onco Labs so that I can see, scientifically, if I have any cancer cells. In the beginning I used to do it every three months, then every six months. This test helps me stay on track and gets me in the right direction if I'm straying. One year, according to this test, my cancer cells were on the rise again. I quickly began to get stricter with myself regarding my diet and cleansing routines, and took the test again in three months. The cancer cells were down.

My cousin, Dr. Rainer, was diagnosed with prostate cancer at the same time I was diagnosed with ovarian cancer. When I went to visit my family in Germany, I would tell him of all the alternative information on health I was learning and how he needed to starve his cancer and cleanse his body. He was a very successful dentist in Germany and his best friend was an oncologist. Rainer would tell me that he was fine. He took the traditional allopathic route for prostate cancer and had surgery to remove his cancer.

Two years after his surgery, he called me in tears that the cancer was back in his lymph nodes. The doctors wanted him on chemotherapy, and being a doctor himself, he knew all the complications of that. He told me that he did not believe (even one little bit) in alternative healing, or what I was doing, but he didn't want chemotherapy, and so alternative was his only other choice. "I'm coming to see you in America," he told me. "You have 18 days to make me believe in alternative healing to treat my cancer." He was being VERY German.

When he came to visit me, it was rough going, to say the least. One morning I caught him eating mango jam on white bread after I had given him strict instructions on the dangers of sugar and starch and white flour. I had explained in detail all I had learned and done during the past two years, and shared all the advice and instructions I had received from the clinics. That wasn't good enough for Rainer. After all, I was just his crazy cousin. I called in a friend of mine, Charles Marble, the former director of Optimum Health Clinic in Naples, to explain to Rainer what food did to the body. Then I took him to the frequency healer in St. Augustine that I had visited. With all this careful explanation from the experts, Rainer transformed from a total nonbeliever of alternative natural healing into a staunch supporter of natural remedies and healthy diet. He immediately began to follow a strict diet and incorporated all the natural remedies he had heard about into his life. Six months later, when they tested his lymph nodes, his cancer had disappeared. Now he helps others learn about natural healing.

I lovingly balance my mind and my body. I now choose thoughts that make me feel good.

~ Louise L. Hay

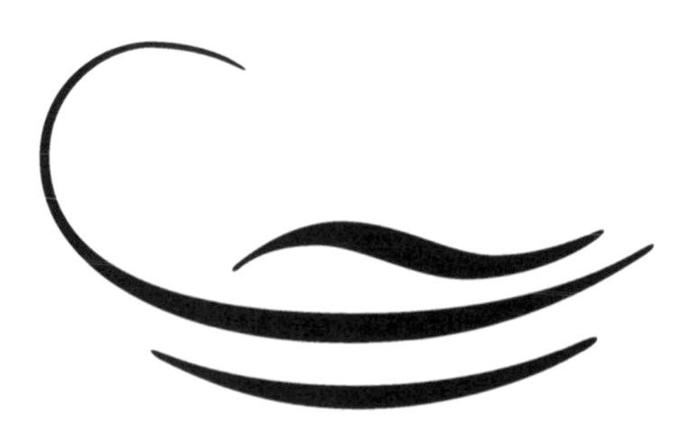

Chapter 5
Emotional Healing

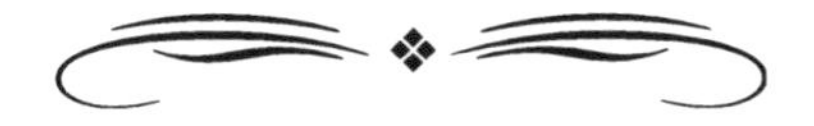

ANOTHER BRANCH OF ALL OF MY alternative learning was "emotional healing." I attended lots of seminars on getting to know myself, clearing my energy, delving into my issues. My friend Yolanda had recommended this Swiss person who did emotional healing and was in Naples, and I went to see her. She asked me "Why do you think, Ursula, that you have let yourself get cancer?" She asked me a lot about my emotions. Being German, all I could think of is, "What the heck do my EMOTIONS have to do with my cancer?" (Little did I know at the time that emotions and their vibrations have everything to do with your health). This Swiss healer did a "psychic operation" on me and gave me Bach remedies to smell. The entire episode was a bit too weird for me at the time. However, I must say that it was the beginning of my realizing that I just may have attracted the cancer to myself in some emotional way. Although I was skeptical during this first experience. I was to take part in many, many, more emotional healings in the future.

Some friends of mine called to let me know they had a book called The Miracles of Natural Healing by Luke Chan on CD. They told me they were also holding a seminar. Once again, I was skeptical but willing to give anything a try. Maybe this "Miracle" business had something to do with it. It turned out to be a two day Qi Gong seminar where you work with good energy in your body.

It felt so good that I found myself doing the Qi Gong exercises all the way home in the car. Yes, while I was driving. I would hold the steering wheel steady with my legs and open my arms to the universe. (I told you I don't waste a minute.) I was pulling in healing energy to my abdominal area. I was lucky I didn't get "pulled over" by the police, however, I was not driving far!

I did these Qi Gong exercises every chance I got for hours throughout the day. But unless you're a very good driver, I would recommend doing them with your feet on the ground, not on a gas pedal.

We had a little graduation ceremony for learning the ten minute daily routine. After the graduation, the instructor told everyone to form a circle. There were about 100 of us. He said that anyone with cancer or any life-threatening illness should stand in the center of the circle, while all the other seminar participants stood around them. Everyone on the outside of the circle directed their energy toward us in the center. This was the first time I had an emotional and mental breakdown. I could not stop crying. An overwhelming feeling of "oh crap" came over me. "OMG, I have cancer." It hit me full force, like all that energy coming at me.

Suddenly I was in touch with my emotions. The biggest one was Fear. This must have been what David felt like when he first caught sight of Goliath.

The next seminar I went to was in Fort Myers, FL. Although this is only the next town over from where I live in Naples, I had a great deal of trouble finding the seminar location. Something was wrong with the directions and they weren't making sense. I called the director of the seminar for help while I was on the road, but still arrived ten minutes late. The moment I passed through the door, I locked horns with the director in a power struggle, like two mountain goats trying to push each other down a different trail. "Oh great" I thought. "What a great way to start an emotional cleansing seminar. I guess I really DO need some work!"

Gradually, with each additional seminar and learning experience, I learned when you have cancer, you need to learn to "let go." I mean **REALLY LET GO**! Enjoy every moment; enjoy every day. But I hadn't learned that yet, and so, I had a slight attitude adjustment to make.

Anyway, we were locked up for four days straight. No phones, no TV, no communication at all with the outside world. The food was all organic and all vegetarian. We worked on ourselves from 9 a.m. until midnight. More than once during this seminar, I would just shake my head in disbelief because of the methods being used to help us release emotions. (Remember, I do have German blood in me.) It was a small group, about 10 of us. I saw everyone releasing emotions and breaking down and crying. So I realized whatever methods were being used were working. We meditated, we did handwriting with our left hand, we learned channeling, we learned to be creative, we wrote poems, we acted out scenarios. After the four days I was exhausted and ready to go home. I had met some interesting people and made some wonderful friends, but I vowed I would never return.

At that seminar, I made a new friend Barbara and some other healers who were aware of the seminar technique and had done it before. They tried to talk me into going to the advanced seminar for another seven days. I didn't want to do it, but I did it as a favor to Barbara. During these seven days, I realized that in order to completely heal myself, I had to clear my body's energetic imprint of all my family patterns and ancestral bad karma. We carry in our bodies all the stories, illnesses, tragedies, pain and grief of our ancestors as energetic imprints in our energy field. The release from these energies truly felt out of this world.

On the first day, we were to be paired up with a partner for the full seven days. By paired up, I mean really stuck next to each other for the full week, mimicking each other's moves. The first day you mimicked your partner, and the next day they mimicked you. Because of my athletic lifestyle, there were people in this seminar that I did not want to be with. The pairing was done randomly through drawings. Luckily, my partner turned out to be a Chinese lady with the same birthday as me, who loved yoga, pilates, and quiet walks. We were perfect for each other because we were on the same wavelength. This turned out to be just what I needed at the time.

What I remember most about this seminar was that we were to chop a block of wood with our hands. The day prior, I had gone swimming with dolphins, so peaceful and calming. Now I had to chop a block of wood with my bare hands. I had been volunteering to do everything first the entire week. This time, when the instructor asked for a volunteer, I stayed quiet. Another girl went first and successfully split the wood with the first try. She was very proud and we all cheered for her. Going first and being successful were just what she needed for her healing. Then someone else went. And then I couldn't hold back any longer. (Remember, "type A" personality!) There was a woman who was in her 70's at the seminar and we all held our breath because she was frail and mild-mannered and we wondered if the wood would split but she walked up front to the block of wood, and going through the moves in slow motion, split the wood before she even touched it. She had split it with her energy - drawing from above and pulling it through the wood. We all sat there staring with our jaws open...

My partner was the last person to go. She had lots of emotions from her relationship with her ex-husband that she needed to release. She could not split the wood. "Don't worry," we all said to her. "Don't worry, it's not meant to be." We comforted her as best as we could, and it turned out that she needed to accept our comfort more than she needed to split the wood. Things all work out that way in life if you are open to realizing what is happening.

Another day we had to jump from the roof of the house into the swimming pool. One woman in attendance was very frightened. She did not know how to swim! We stood below for 1 ½ hours encouraging her. Finally she jumped. She cried and laughed and was very excited because she had conquered her fear, and we all cried and laughed right with her.

We also did a very revealing standing meditation. Starting with our partners, toe to toe, we just stared into each others eyes. There were six outside the circle and six inside. After each meeting, the whole circle shifted one person down so we all got to stare in everyone's eyes.

When my partner and I stared into each others eyes, I saw myself as a young Chinese girl walking the rice fields and having fun with her. It lasted for about three to five minutes. It was incredible. When I shifted to the next girl, as soon as we locked eyes, we started laughing and laughing and couldn't stop. We instinctively knew that in a past life, we must have been very good friends. When Ruby (the older lady who split the wood with her energy) looked into my eyes, I saw her as my mother in a past life and cried. Next in line was a man who was known as a healer. He came closer into "my space" than the others had and had a very strong stare. I stared right back and felt myself getting taller and stronger and had a strange certainty that we were in Egyptian times. We were reliving a power struggle.

I had a different experience with each person. I felt I had lived a past life with each person. It was a wonderfully healing experience to be with such a group of people and feel so close. Every night we sang a song together and hugged each other. It was a special connection with a special grouping of souls.

I'm telling you all this so you can see what an incredible experience this was for me who had been so dogmatic my entire life. Before these experiences, I had very little exposure to spiritual or emotional events. The closest foray had been hypnosis. I had wanted to learn two or three languages at the same time and a hypnotist offered to put me under. I laughed at him and told him it would never happen, but within an instant I was under. He said I spoke in a different tongue and he wanted me to come back, but I never wanted to see him again. So the experiences during this seminar were extraordinary for me. It proved to me that there are forces beyond what we can see that affect our health and well-being.

The last night of the seven day seminar, we were hypnotized with music and energy so we would go into a space with past lives. Everyone had a past life experience except for me. I had the sensation and visuals of an eagle flying free for the entire session. I loved it.

I went to another seminar along these lines in the middle of New York near SoHo. It was a six day Shamanistic seminar in a Buddhist retreat center. We had to walk around barefoot all the time. I remember they served a GREAT breakfast (lots of organic fruit and vegetables), and there was lots and lots of meditation. It was led by a female who used to have a career in advertising. One day she had gone to Peru and learned healing and emotional release workshops from Shamans. It changed her life.

My friend Judy (from the clinics in Mexico) met me there. It was a very mind-opening experience. There are many different versions of healing in this world and I urge you to be courageous enough to explore until you find the one that works for you. Not everything works for everybody. And most of us need to attack our healing from more than one angle.

Music is also a form of healing. My Oncologist friend told me that the song "The Flight of the Bumble Bee" by Nikolai Rimsky-Korsakov has a frequency in the music that works on cancer. Specifically ovarian cancer so I played that CD every night before I went to bed.

I felt a lot of different shifts going on with regard to my mental and emotional state as I took seminar after seminar on emotional releasing and continued learning about energetic's. My journey of healing was not just about taking the right pills or herbs or vitamins or shakes. It was about the frequencies of my emotions and mental attitude too. Everything is connected, so cleansing the physical, mental, emotional, and spiritual body is a must. Just like earth, fire, water, air, and wood. They all affect each other constantly.

In Chicago I saw a Chinese herbalist. It took me three weeks to get the appointment. The first thing I had to do was show him my tongue. He would shake his head and mumble "too red; serious illness." I told him about the chemo/ radiation and he said "No chemo - No radiation." He gave me stuff to drink that was absolutely awful. He told me to sell everything I owned and quit my job or I would never get rid of my cancer. Yeah, right.

Within a year I made the decision to sell everything I had in Chicago and start fresh in Naples, Florida. I left all my "bad vibes" behind. All my stress and everything I knew were now behind me.

It's really YOUR path. Everyone is different. But I want to suggest, educate, and give you choices. Different methods work for different people. It's essential that you learn as much as you can and see what works for you.

I had never told my mother that I had cancer. She was elderly and still lived in Germany. Since there was a history of cancer in my family, I did not want to worry her. My brother, Gerhard, wanted to prove how German and tough my mother was so he persuaded me to tell my mother some years after. I said, "Mother, I had cancer" and she stopped me in my tracks. "Do you still have cancer?" She asked sharply. "No." "Then why are we talking about it?" She said with a dismissive wave of her hand. That was the end of our conversation about cancer.

No Fears, No worries. This is really important. It used to be whenever I had a pain somewhere I would think, "Oh my God!" Now, you need to get rid of your fears. No worries. Healing is a commitment for LIFE never to attract cancer again.

It is so important to have an open mind!

The next story is my cousin who did not believe in alternative healing at all. He also did not believe that nutrition mattered in regard to cancer.

I am so pleased that my cousin Rainer jumped through his fear of doom. He was finally ready to open his mind, listening, and learning how you can heal the body naturally by using alternative remedies.

I am important. I count. I now care for and nourish myself with love and with joy. I allow others the freedom to be who they are. We are all safe and free.

~ Louise L. Hay

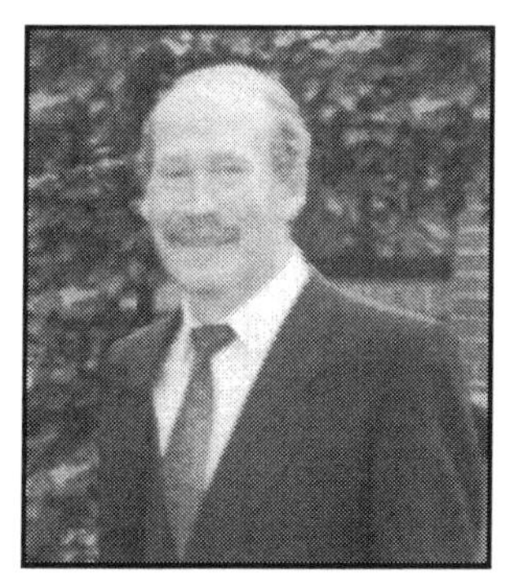

Dr. Rainer Merkel

Chapter 6
My Cousin's Story
By Dr. Rainer Merkel

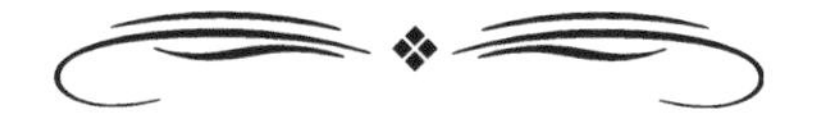

DURING A PREVENTATIVE MEDICAL checkup in 1999, which I had not taken advantage of for years, doctors found that my PSA value had increased. After a biopsy and CT imaging, they found a prostate carcinoma that had already spread into my prostate capsule. I was 54 years old at that time, had a large dental practice, and was rather stressed due to my intense focus at work.

I had a harmonious environment with my wife and three sons and was very athletic with numerous activities, which I thought provided for an excellent balance. I was pretty buff, athletic, and actually felt rather fit. I neither smoke nor do I consume any significant amounts of alcohol. I have a balanced diet, proper nutrition, and take loads of vitamins. Up until then, I had never wasted a single thought on cancer.

The information that was available to me on types of surgery was unmistakable. From an orthodox medicine point of view, only radical surgery including the removal of lymph nodes was an option, which I had done immediately. During surgery, the urethra was also shortened and reconnected to the base of the bladder. Following a three week stay at the hospital, I underwent rehabilitation treatment to strengthen my pelvic floor muscles including the accompanying improvement of my continence. However, no mention was made about any lifestyle changes.

I was discharged from rehab as being cured. After a six month break, I gradually resumed my activities at the dentist office. At the same time, my cousin Ursula visited and reported her own serious battle against cancer. I was amazed when she shared the positive experiences she had after a rather difficult course of disease while using alternative methods of treatment. Because of the risk of a relapse, she advised me on how to change my life: avoid stress, change my nutrition, and strengthen my immune system. "Why did you get cancer," was her important question. "Only a weak immune system will allow that to happen."

However, as an orthodox medical practitioner, I did not dwell much on Ursula's suggestions even though I frequently felt tired, unwell and unable to work under pressure. During a subsequent examination in 2001 my PSA value had increased again. The CT images showed a relapse in the shape of significantly enlarged lymph nodes.

The physicians advised me to undergo comprehensive surgery including the removal of all lymph tracts and lymph nodes up to the mediastinum. This surgical intervention would have massively compromised my quality of life. I was shocked about this message and filled with fear. After consulting with Ursula and my wife, who also was more open to alternative methods of healing, I agreed to immediately fly to Florida and use Ursula's recommendations through her own experiences.

In Florida, I was counseled by an interdisciplinary team consisting of nutritionists, psychologists and physiotherapists on the complex interrelations in the body. Together, we retrieved my patient history.

An examination lasting several days by Dr. Jack Garvy in St. Augustine revealed, among other things, degenerated cells indicating cancer, viruses (due to protracted flu), fungi, bacteria and significant stress due to chemicals and disinfectants from my activities at my dental practice.

During intensive discussions, we became very familiar with each other. I gradually felt that the disease was a part of me that I myself could realize and that I could and must learn to deal with. A frequency treatment recommended by Dr. Garvy combined with Essiac Tea and a consistent change in my food habits (no sugar!) already yielded improved values during our stay in Florida. Sugar is an ideal food for cancer cells. I had to quit drinking coffee, alcohol, nicotine, wheat flour, milk products of any type, meat, sausage, etc. It was rather tedious to find foods free from chemical additives, preservatives, yeast, sugar... basically only organic foods. The same applies to fruits and vegetables too.

I learned how important and critical an alkaline nutritional diet is, because cancer cells prefer to settle in acidic environments. Also educating myself about water and salt became very important for me. At this point, I was consuming three liters of pure, non-carbonated water a day, and using sea salt or Himalayan salt. I developed a strong awareness about our food and our environment.

This is how I lost my fear of cancer, because I was able to actively perceive myself. After changing my entire life, giving up my practice and the insights gained on nutrition and frequencies, I soon felt better. Regular CT examinations and blood work showed a significant reduction of the lymph nodes, to the physicians' surprise.

I have AMAS blood work done on a regular basis in Florida that shows any type of cancer in its earliest stages. I am so grateful to my wife, my cousin Ursula, Dr. Jack Garvy, Charles Marble, and all the alternative practitioners in Florida. Their support allowed me to lead my current life.

Experiences come and
go however; my love
for myself is constant.
~ Louise L. Hay

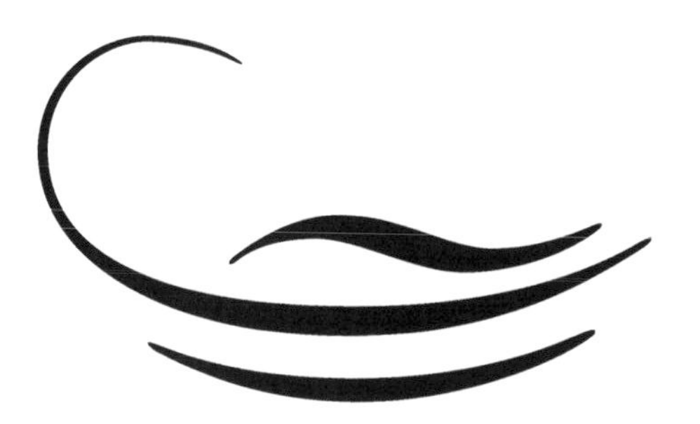

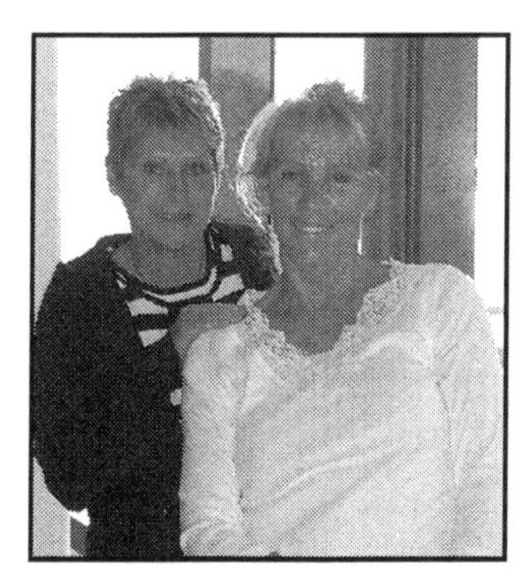

Judy Sabers (left) and Ursula Kaiser

Chapter 7
My Best Friend Judy Sabers' Story - SEEKING WELLNESS

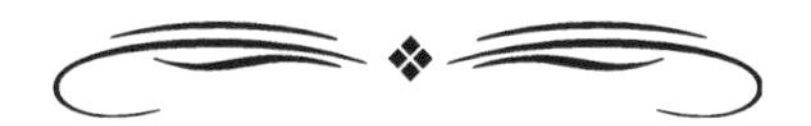

I WANT TO THANK JUDY FOR COMING into my life and extending her friendship at a crucial time in our lives. Your friendship enabled me to open up and share our journey to health and wellness. Being able to communicate with you at any time on the phone, sharing the latest information we found, our many healing trips we did together, and all the emotional seminars we participated in made the journey so empowering. Your friendship through our healing was the biggest blessing and gift of all. I cannot imagine what this journey would have been without your loving support. We will always motivate each other to stay on track. I am grateful for Judy's insight and sharing her story, as follows, SEEKING WELLNESS!

In June of 1999, my world changed. After having a "suspicious" mammogram in 1998, I had been scheduled for mammograms and checkups every six months. Each time, several views were taken and examined. In June of 1999, the radiologist came out from behind her hiding place and told me that I needed to see a surgeon as soon as possible. There were calcifications present that indicated DCIS, ductal carcinoma in situ. By the time I got home, there was a message from a surgeon's office saying I had an appointment at 8:30 the following morning. (As a side note here, research has now shown that radiation from mammograms can increase a women's chance of getting breast cancer.)

Then it began. I felt like I had totally lost control of my life. A biopsy indicated problems; and since the DCIS was widespread, I was told that a radical mastectomy was the answer and should totally take care of the problem. No chemo or radiation should be necessary.

The "overnight" surgery was scheduled for July 7, 1999. I would be able to go home that next morning. But when noon came and I hadn't been released, I started asking questions. The doctor would be here shortly. His news was unexpected.

Not only had DCIS been present but so had two more tumors: one ERPR positive and the other ERPR negative. The cancer was rated Stage IIB. Stage IIB describes invasive breast cancer in which the tumor is larger than 2 cm but no larger than 5 cm and has spread to the auxiliary lymph nodes. How could that be? I had done mammograms every six months, exactly as the doctor had recommended. How did it get this advanced? Lymph node involvement meant chemo and radiation—six months of it. And later tests indicated a positive HER2/Neu gene which further complicated the situation. The HER2/Neu indicates an aggressive, fast growing cancer that almost always returns within three years and is unstoppable.

The next three weeks were a series of doctor appointments, surgeon appointments, and tests of all kinds to make sure I was "healthy" enough to withstand surgery, chemo, and radiation. Pamphlets and booklets littered the table. And did I want to do reconstruction? Read this book about your choices. A wig had to be fitted and ordered; bras and a prosthesis had to be purchased.

Three weeks after surgery, I walked into the infusion room for the first chemo, after getting a portacath installed earlier that morning. A friend who had gone through chemo two years earlier sat at my side during the three hour infusion of

Adriomyicin and Cytoxin, and took me home. Then the fun began. The anti-nausea meds didn't work. Two days later, I ended up back in the hospital from dehydration. At that point I decided that the treatment was worse than the disease; there had to be a better way. Fourteen days after that one chemo, my hair started falling out in gobs so I got my head shaved. With tears streaming down my face, the reality really hit home!

After that first chemo, I immediately started doing research on the Internet and bought three books that consumed my days. I knew that the next chemo was scheduled in three weeks, and I had to make a decision by then. I read about alternative products and treatments and the clinics that offered them. After narrowing down choices, I selected Tijuana, Mexico, operated by an American doctor who drove over the border from California, to do what he couldn't do in the US.

I walked into the Mexican clinic exactly three weeks after that first and only chemo. Had I been on vacation, I would have thought it was great! A courtyard with trees and plants surrounded a pool. But instead of vacationers, there were some very sick looking people occupying the chairs.

I was greeted by a group of doctors and nurses. The doctor assigned to my case assessed my situation and developed a protocol for me. Their strategy was based on strengthening the immune system so it could fight the cancer. I got cancer because of an immune system that didn't do its job, so let's get it built up and working!

For the next 3 weeks, I had daily IV infusions of nutrients including high dose Vitamin B and C and Dioxichlor which is an oxygen supplement. FYI - pathogens cannot live in an oxygenated environment. I took Laetrile which is a Vitamin B 17, known as a cancer killer. I also did a few doses of hematoxilan, nicknamed The Red Devil, the closest to a chemo agent that the clinic used but not nearly as toxic as the agents used in the United States.

This clinic treated mind, body, and spirit. The food was organic, mostly raw, and included a variety of vegetables and salads with a healthy vinegar and oil dressing. Only once did we have fish, and it was delicious! Fresh green juices were served daily. Only limited fruit was served, because we were told, sugar feeds cancer, and even though fruit contains a natural sugar, it's still sugar. Those cancer cells do a little jig when they get a taste of that sugar coming down the pipe! We were told to avoid anything sweet and anything white or made from something white — bread, rice, potatoes, anything made from white flour. No dairy products were offered. I learned so much about healthy eating from the information provided by the clinic, and I still continue that quest to learn more about living a healthy lifestyle. I had asked an oncologist in the US after surgery what I should be eating. His reply was, "Anything that tastes good to you." How totally wrong that answer was!

At the clinic, we were offered acupuncture, an age-old practice based on Traditional Chinese Medicine, to clear blockages from the meridians, the energy flow or Chi running through our bodies. When energy blockages develop, disease follows. Deep breathing exercises were encouraged. Most of us shallow breathe and therefore don't get good oxygen into the blood stream. A psychologist held small group discussions and helped us grasp and deal with our situations and encouraged us to talk about our fears and thoughts. The mind is a powerful tool for healing, so guided imagery was offered. We used our imaginations to visualize the cancer being eaten by a little Pac-Man or any other image that we choose. Meditation was encouraged as was movement and exercise if at all possible.

After three weeks, I went home with a renewed pledge to beat this thing. I changed diet and lifestyle. I feel healthier than ever. Many people describe their journey through cancer as a journey through hell. My journey was different. Because of the people I've met and the things I've learned. I wouldn't change anything. I'm one of the fortunate ones.

It was at this clinic that I met Ursula, due to a wrong number! In Chicago, both Ursula and her friend, Vanda, were also dealing with cancer. The first day at the clinic, the phone in my room rang. No one knew I was there! Who could it be? Vanda, who was calling another patient, was patched through to my room by mistake. But since I was on the line, she decided to ask questions about how my treatment was going and said she and a friend were trying to choose a clinic. Four days later, Ursula and Vanda walked into my room. That was 12 years ago. Ursula and I have remained close friends since that first visit and get together every year. We've done a lot of healing together, including changes in diet and lifestyle, cleansing, reiki, frequency healing based on Rife technology, and attending an energy medicine workshop with Donna Eden, to name a few. We continue to do regular detoxifications and cleanses (coffee enemas, green drinks, juice fasts, herbal teas, Essiac tea, and Jusuru, a nutrient dense juice drink.) We both laugh about the "stuff" we've taken, some horrible tasting, and the things we've done, all in the name of healing! And it's worked for us! When you know what the option is, it becomes much easier to "down" some of those less desirable tasting drinks, do cleanses, and heal the emotions!

Now, twelve years later, I no longer feel it's necessary to go out of the country to find good treatment. There have been so many breakthroughs in the last decade. There are excellent clinics within the United States as well as great supplements and healing tools, including lasers, light pens, and Rife technologies available to anyone who seeks them out. To those of you who are traveling through your journey toward health and wellness, I commend you for your strength, commitment, and resolution to do what you know in your gut and heart are right for you. It's not easy to buck the system, if that becomes your choice of treatment. Listen to your inner self. It will guide you in the direction you are meant to travel.

I release the pattern in me that
attracted this experience.
I create only good in my life.
~ Louise L. Hay

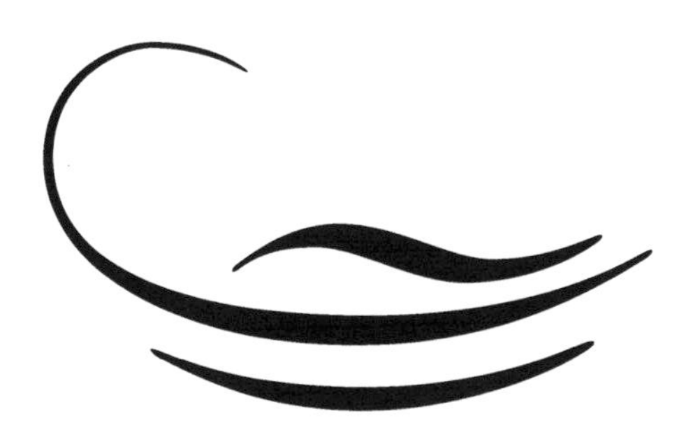

We are each responsible
for all of our experiences.

Every thought we think is creating our future.

The point of power is always
in the present moment.

Everyone suffers from self-hatred and guilt.

The bottom line for everyone is
"I'm not good enough."

It's only a thought, and a
thought can be changed.

We create every so-called illness in the body.

Resentment, criticism, and guilt are the most
damaging patterns.

Releasing resentment will dissolve even cancer.

We must release the past and forgive everyone.

We must be willing to begin
to learn to love ourselves.

Self-approval and self-acceptance
in the now are the keys to positive change.

When we really love ourselves,
everything in our life works.

~ Louise L. Hay

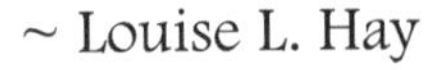

Chapter 8
Consciousness and Cancer
By Noel Inniss

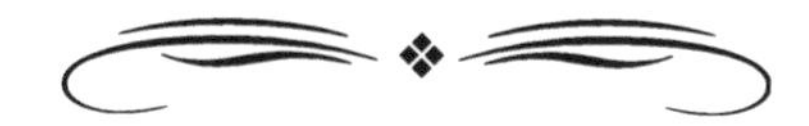

WHAT IS CONSCIOUSNESS?
Consciousness is defined in the dictionary as knowing what is around you. What is not explored is the idea of consciousness that makes up how we perceive and who we think we are.

There are basically two types of consciousness. There is natural consciousness within the body. For instance, the liver has to have the consciousness of a liver to perform the duties of the liver. The pancreas has its own consciousness to carry out its duties as a pancreas which is different from the liver.

This is known as the natural consciousness unique to that organ, endocrine or body part. There are different consciousnesses that form a network of communication which carry out billions of functions in the body at any given moment. Each organ, endocrine, and body part has a natural consciousness. There is also pathological consciousness which creates disease. Consciousness is still not understood by most of us, so let me try to bring more awareness to this matter.

Consciousness we can say is made up of thoughts or concepts. So what is a thought? A thought is an impulse of energy and information. It is non matter. And every time there is a thought matter formed, a neuropeptide, first messenger molecule, goes to receptors in the brain. The brain transfers it to the cells, and the cells automatically respond. Even if you're sleeping and dreaming that someone is chasing you with a baseball bat, if you awake you'll find your heart pounding; you are sweating. Your cells are responding even though you're sleeping. If you have a weak heart you can have a heart attack in your sleep and not even be aware of it. Twenty-four / seven your cells are being bombarded with impulses from the mind and have not evolved to the point where they can rationalize. They cannot take a joke, as Dr. Deepak Chopra would say. We will survive, you know. It's just the quality of life. So in part consciousness is our thoughts formed by our conditioning and experiences that makes up our belief system. It also makes up who we think we are or how we should act. It is said that 95% of the reasons we visit the doctors offices are stress related. Stress is only how one perceives what he is experiencing at that moment. Perception is what you think about something, which are your thoughts. Stress is not the number one killer in the world; thoughts are. The thoughts that make up your belief system can be the number one killer in the world. So if we're experiencing disease, it would seem important to address what our cells have been experiencing throughout our lifetime.

Louise Hay's book, "You Can Heal Your Body", outlines the metaphysical basis behind cancer. It is deep hurt, long-standing resentment, grieving, and carrying around hatred. The cells in our body respond to impulses without question. Surely we must realize how important it is to investigate what we think since what we think is also who we think we are.

Ideas and concepts are not the problem. The damage occurs with the level of involvement and emotional attachment to them. As we use concepts to communicate and interact with the world, which are the proper uses of them, we can be a little more aware of how the cells are responding. This is also relative to the level of emotional involvement with them. This can also be a measure on how much one loves oneself.

There would not be any long standing resentment or any carrying around hatred if we understood more about the natural consciousness of the body and which part we want to do the processing for us. If you guessed the heart, then hooray! The heart is the central organizer and processer. Energy that comes to us is best processed through the heart. The heart will produce the appropriate concept; compassion, forgiveness, love, etc. If the processing is fear, it lands in the kidneys or if frustration and anger, it will affect the liver.

Healing implies wholeness and wholeness implies a totality of perspectives. We cannot choose one over another and expect it to work in all situations. To experience wholeness we must be open to all points of view. If we trained ourselves to process all our experiences through our hearts, to be aware of love all the time, we would exist on a very high level of consciousness indeed.

The likes of great ones like Buddha and Jesus. It is important that we become aware of the thoughts that permeate our being. They form the consciousness and belief systems that our cells respond to. If thought comes before matter, then consciousness is before physical manifestation. Proper energy with regard to the intake of foods is important. Cleanse the body often, and learn to master how to interact with the world from your heart center. It is at this time that our cells will be receiving happier and healthier messages.

In the final healthy analysis...

"LOVE IS ALL THERE IS!"

Noel is a healer, tennis pro, massage therapist and so much more
239-595-7676 • Noelinniss@yahoo.com

Seek the gift in all that happens
and you shall find peace within.
~ Unknown

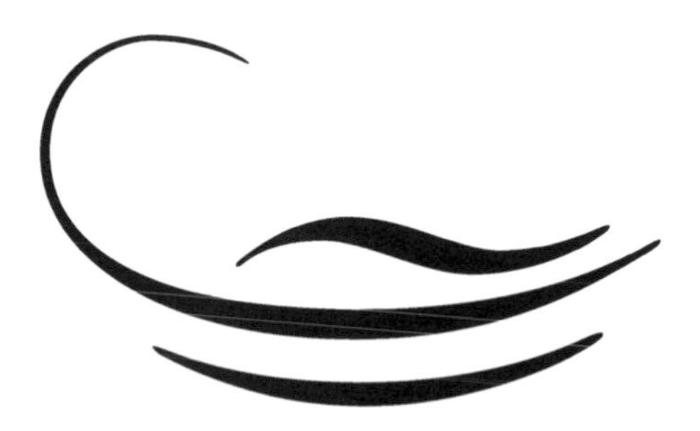

Chapter 9

Losing A Loved One to Cancer

By Joyce A. Pellegrini
Certified Biofeedback Practitioner
Stress Management Coach Using Energy

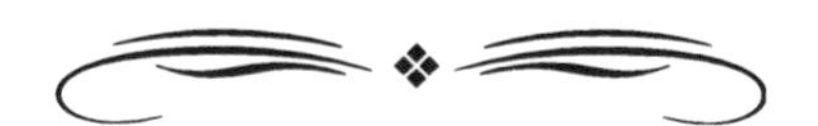

ONE DAY I WAS SITTING AT THE CAR wash waiting for my car to be completed when my phone rang; it was my sister Gina. She asked "Where are you?" I could tell from her voice that something was wrong and knew it was not good! I said "What is wrong?" She then started to cry and tell me that my baby brother, Perry, was diagnosed with stage 4 stomach cancer. I could not believe what I was hearing. I also remembered my brother complaining all the time about acid reflux. He was popping *Tums* like candy. I kept telling him to go to the doctor, but he had no insurance at that time and had just started a new job!

The only person that had cancer in our family was my Nonna, my dad's mother, who had breast cancer early in life and had one breast removed. However, Nonna lived until she was 96 years old so I knew Perry could win his battle too.

So after speaking with my sister, I went home, packed up my little two seater car, my dog Rocky, and my office and drove home from Florida to Chicago to assist my brother in fighting this ugly disease. I knew he was tough and he could beat the odds. He was a Pellegrini, we are fighters!

I had been in search of natural healing modalities due to my own medical issues and was sick of taking pills that did not help. One weekend, I was visiting Ursula and had the pleasure of meeting Barbara Ellis at the beach and was fascinated by what Barbara did professionally. I always meet interesting people hanging with Ursula and knew she keeps up with the latest and greatest healing tools that are available. Ursula is the only person I know that truly walks her talk. I will admit I have never seen Ursula put anything unhealthy in her mouth and I understand why.

Barbara educated me on her quantum biofeedback device, and I was so intrigued that I booked a session with her the following day. The SCIO was able to detect how stress affected my mental, emotional, physical, and spiritual body. My session with Barbara blew me away; she not only told me a few physical issues that I had that were chronic, but also identified that my stress was really due to my mental and emotional health. I had extreme suppressed anger. The machine also said that I never spoke my truth, which explains my thyroid being taken out at the early age of 17. This was why I had been an insomniac for over 20 years, due to all my emotions running like a rat on a wheel in my head, and I was never able to communicate them effectively due to fear of expressing myself. I did three more sessions with Barbara and knew that I had found my next career - helping others like me understand how stress truly causes disease. I wanted to empower people to claim back their lives through education. This story about me is important because it will tell you what I learned when I went home to help my brother fight his battle against cancer.

Through my studies and asking Ursula what to do, I began juicing every day for Perry. I removed the microwave, Teflon pans, plastics, and any other toxic materials in Perry's kitchen. No more junk foods! I bought all organic veggies, and I went to the best natural wellness store and bought him Essiac Tea and vitamins that I was told to get to help fight the symptoms of the radical chemo and radiation he was going to undertake. My sister Gina took him to an Amish healer who told Perry it would be the hardest fight of his life but he would live if he totally detoxed the body. He said he would do whatever it took. I did not need to hear anything else. I was on it!

Perry was given a port for the chemo so I took him to the hospital three to four times a week for his treatments. Perry had stomach cancer and he could barely swallow. He was having a hard time eating and drinking. When I spoke to the doctor, he did not want Perry to do anything other than the trial drugs he was given in this program. The doctor kept telling him to eat whatever he wanted as long as he ate something. My intuition told me that the cancer was not just in his stomach. I believed it was everywhere in his body. Perry was in so much pain, he could not sleep at night so they put him on Ambien to sleep. I would give him a massage every night to try and calm him but he could not relax. I know how we Pellegrinis are and knew my baby brother ran those words through his mind over and over again "You have 7 months to live." We did, however, fire his first doctor immediately. She had no bed side manner, was cold so we wanted nothing to do with her.

Perry was a walking time bomb ready to explode at any time. He was so angry and exhausted, he did not want anyone around him including me. Prior to my getting to Perry's house, I had just purchased my SCIO device and was beginning the training process. I decided I would begin to do a biofeedback session on him every other day, due to his life threatening illness. I would do anything I could to help him fight his battle. Every day I would disappear into the living room to began to teach myself how to operate the new device I had purchased while he sat in front of the TV. My own journey began. You see as I looked into my brother's face, I saw a mirror reflection of myself... but my emotions were deep seated and suppressed – **not good**!

So the reason I am writing a chapter in this book is to share what I learned from this experience showing how your mental and emotional health drives physical illnesses in the body. Every emotion my brother felt showed up on the device – fear, anger, resentment, desire for things to be different, religious conflict, resistance to change, worry, anxiety, just to name a few. What this taught me was that negative emotions will cause disease in the body, especially when you are not eating a clean and healthy diet. My brother drank beer every night, smoked pot, ate fast foods, worked in a high stress career, was fighting a custody battle, and felt resentment toward the woman who was keeping him from his only son. With so many toxic things going on in his physical body, his immune system was not strong enough to fight his battle.

Perry was told he had seven months to live, and he died seven months from his diagnosis. No one should ever tell you how much time you have to live. Our minds are very powerful. When you do not fight ill thoughts, you then become them. It is that simple. I learned this saying at a seminar… **CHANGE YOUR THOUGHTS – CHANGE YOUR LIFE**. It took me several months to truly embrace that statement, but I found how true it was in my own life! **HEALTH GOES WHERE ENERGY FLOWS.** It is truly that simple, but our minds make it so much more complex when pride and ego get in the way.

Through the loss of my brother, I received a new lease on life. I do not drink, I exercise daily, I realign my spirit to have faith in a higher power GOD, and I ask for his blessings on a daily basis. I have been blessed to know Ursula Kaiser and I watch how she inspires people daily with her knowledge of how to detoxify the body, keep that vessel clean for a long, vibrant, and healthy life, so you may live an abundant life.

Please forgive all who have hurt you, please forgive yourself for all of your past mistakes, know that you are loved from above, detoxify the body from all of its impurities with the cleanses that are in this book (they work,) have only loving and supportive people around you, watch funny movies only, laugh as much as you can, reconnect with mother nature, put your feet in the sand, take salt baths, talk to the animals around you, journal every day and write down all the things you are grateful for. If you are angry at someone, write them a letter. Let out all the negativity then burn it outside and let it go. This is a very healing process and will allow you to say the words unspoken to allow the healing process to begin. Remember to listen to beautiful music like **FLIGHT OF THE BUMBLEBEE**, and know that you are not alone. We are all here to cheerlead you on to **KICK BUTT IN YOUR FIGHT FOR HEALTH AND WELLNESS NATURALLY**.

Be Blessed and We Hope to Hear From You and How You Are Winning Your Fight! If you would like additional information, please contact Joyce at 813-545-8687 or email: joycepellegrini@gmail.com

Change is the natural law of my life.
I welcome change. I am willing to change.
I choose to change my thinking. I choose
to change my words I use. I move from
the old to the new with ease and with joy.
It is easier for me to forgive than
I thought. Forgiving makes me feel
free and light. It is with joy that I learn
to love myself more and more. The more
resentment I release, the more love I have
to express. Changing my thoughts makes
me feel good. I am learning to choose to
make today a pleasure to experience.
All is well in my world.
~ Louise L. Hay

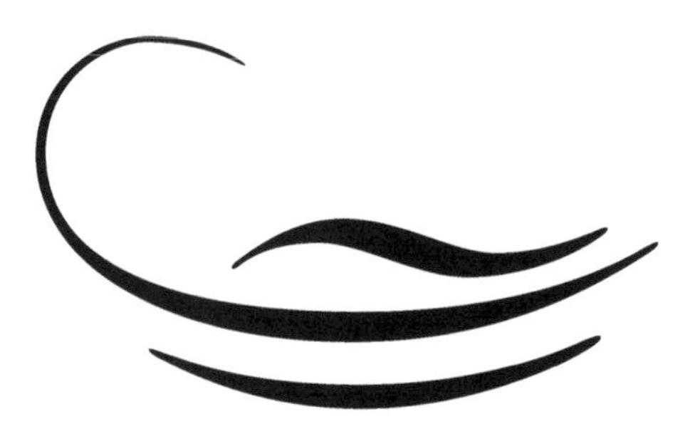

PART 2

HOW TO FIGHT A WINNING BATTLE

I've dedicated the second part of my book to various protocols that have helped me and others to not only stop our cancer from progressing, but eliminate it, and prevent it from coming back.

I will suggest several books that I have read. Please remember that new books are being written every day as one person after another decides to stand up and share their knowledge. I highly suggest you work with a health care provider that you trust. But, please do your own research. It's your health. Take charge.

The freedom of an illness is that YOU are in charge of it. We attract things into our lives, and if we don't like what we've attracted, we can change it. You decide what is right for you.

Communicate with clarity.
Enjoy Heaven and Earth stay in the present moment. Be immune to other's opinions. Replace fear with love (self love). Ignore the opinion of others. Love and respect yourself. Let go of self-judgment and blame. Surrender and let go of the past. Love and nurture your body.

~ Don Miguel Ruiz

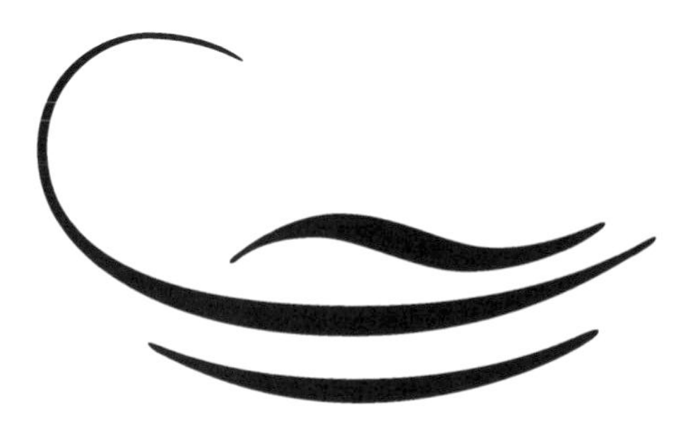

Chapter 10
How To Stop Your Cancer From Progressing!

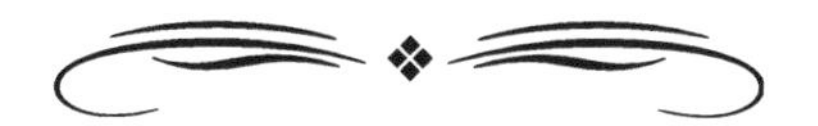

WHILE YOU ARE DECIDING EXACTLY which path you want to take for your healing, you MUST immediately stop your cancer from progressing. Therefore, you must stop giving it the things that it needs to survive.

That means no more sugar. No more starch. No alcohol. No more toxins. No more acidic foods. No more fruit (for right now). Fruit has a high content of sugar, and for right now, we're not going to give that cancer ANYTHING that will help it grow. You absolutely must change your diet.

I am protected by Divine Love. I am always safe and secure. I am willing to grow up and take responsibility for my life. I forgive others, and I now create my own life the way I want it. I am safe.

~ Louise L. Hay

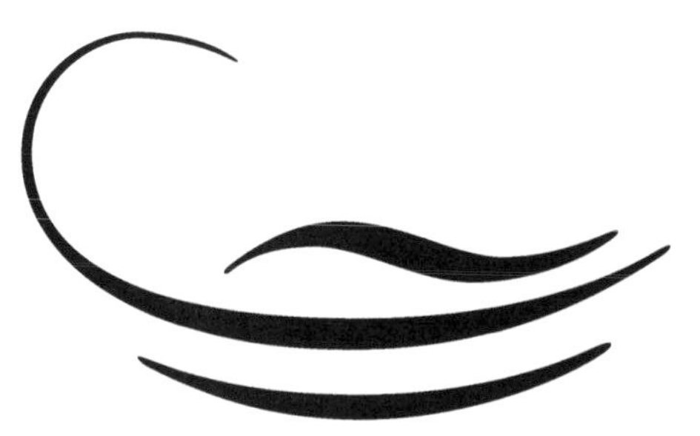

Chapter 11

The Acid - Alkaline Concept

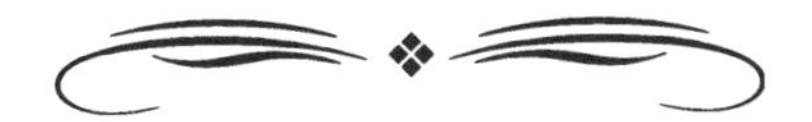

CANCER GROWS IN AN ACIDIC environment, and the typical American diet is predominantly acid forming. Besides, we are always producing acid compounds in our bodies just through normal daily human functions. It is very important to eat an abundance of alkaline forming foods (while limiting the acidic foods) in order to maintain a healthy acid-alkaline balance. On a scale of 0 - 14, 7 is neutral. Our blood needs to be at 7.4 to maintain proper alkalinity. We can accomplish this by eating the proper foods, deep breathing, rest, fresh air, happy thoughts and relaxation. These all contribute to alkalizing our blood.

If your body has an overload of acids and cannot neutralize them, they will nest in the joints and tissues creating pain and disease. Properly balancing your acid/alkaline foods is essential to supporting your immune system.

Simply put, an acidic body contains excess hydrogen. In order to balance it must combine with available oxygen to form water, neutralizing the excess. The result of an acidic body is a constant depletion of internal oxygen!! Cancer cannot thrive in oxygen. If you're depleting your oxygen on a constant basis, you are making it easier for your cancer to survive.

DIET

In the beginning you must eliminate immediately all sugar, starches, yeast, and fruit. Here's a listing of acidic/alkaline foods so you can start avoiding what's bad and give your body what it needs.

Alkaline Forming Foods 80% of Diet (These Are Good)

Fruits

Apples

Apricots

Avocados

Bananas (ripe)

Berries (all)

Cantaloupe

Cherries

Currants

Dates

Figs

Grapes

Mangoes

Melons (all)

Olives (fresh)

Papayas

Raisins

Lemons & Limes

Citrus fruits are acidic, yet because of their high calcium content they produce an alkaline effect during the digestive process. People can experience citrus fruits as acid or as alkaline.

Vegetables

Asparagus, Ripe

Aubergine

Avocados

Beets and Tops

Broccoli

Cabbage Red & White

Carrots

Celery

Chard

Chicory

Chives

Cowslip

Cucumber

Cauliflower

Dandelion Greens

Dill

Alkaline Forming (Good) Foods continued

Dock - Green
Dulse - Seaweed
Endive
Garlic
Green Beans
Kale
Lettuces
Lima Beans
Mushroom - Chitake / Portabello
Parsnips
Peppers, Yellow & Red
Potatoes (All) Radish
Pumpkin
Soybeans
Sorrel
Spinach
Spring Greens
Squash
String Beans
Swede
Turnips and Tops
Watercress

Dairy Products
Acidophilus
Buttermilk
Milk (raw)
Whey
Goats Milk Yogurt

Flesh Foods
None

Cereals
Millet
Corn - Green 1st 24 Hrs

Nuts
Almonds
Chestnuts
Herbal Teas
Honey
Fresh Coconuts
Wheatgrass and Other Sprouted Grasses
Sprouted Whole Grains
Sprouted Legumes
Soaked or Sprouted Nuts and their By-Products

Alkaline Forming (Good) Foods continued

Soaked or Sprouted Seeds and their By-Products

Algaes and Sea Vegetables

Enzymes

Miscellaneous

Agar-Agar

Alfalfa Products

Apple Cider Vinegar

Alkalizers

Cold Showers

Love

Laughter

Fresh Air

Beaches / Negative Ions

Easy way to Alkaline the Body – **GOOD OLD FASHION BAKING SODA REMEDY**

- Internally – Aluminum free baking soda – **BOB'S RED MILL** 1 – 2 teaspoons in water is a powerful alkalizer 2 times a day.
- For **Skin Cancer** – make a paste with the Baking Soda and Water put on area over night – healing remedy that works.

Acid Forming Foods 20% of Diet (These Are Bad)

FRUITS

Citrus

Chestnuts Roasted

Coconuts (Fresh)

All Preserves, Jellies/ Jams - Canned, Sugared, Glazed, Fruit

Green Bananas

Cranberries

Plums

Prunes and Prune Juice

Olives, All Pickles

VEGETABLES

Asparagus Tips

Beans (All)

Brussel Sprouts

Chickpeas

Lentils

Onions

Peanuts

Rhubarb

Tomatoes

DAIRY PRODUCTS

Butter

Cheese (All)

Cream - Ice Cream

Custard

Milk (Boiled, Cooked, Dried, Pasteurized, Canned)

FLESH FOODS

All Meat and Fowl

Shellfish

Gelatin

Gravies

CEREALS

All Flour Products

Buckwheat

Barley

Breads (All Kinds)

Cakes

Corn (All Kinds)

Crackers/Biscuits Doughnuts

Dumplings

Pasta (All)

Noodles

Oatmeal

Pies & Pastries

Rice

Rye-Crisp

Nuts

All Nuts (more so if roasted)

Coconut - Dried

Peanuts

Neutral

Oils - Olive, Corn, Cottenseed, Soy, Sesame

Miscellaneous

Alcohol

Candy

Cocoa

Chocolate

Coca-Cola - All Sodas

Condiments

Dressings

Sauces

Drugs (Aspirin, etc.)

Eggs (Especially Whites)

Ginger – Preserve

Flavorings

Marmalades

Preservatives

Corn Flour

Tobacco

Vinegars – Rice, Wine, etc.

Acidifiers

Lack of Sleep

Overwork

Worry

Tension

Anger

Jealousy

Resentment

Acidity Remedies

Lemon Juice w/1 Tsp. Cider Vinegar; Add Hot Water & Honey

Calcium

Natural Phos. Tissue Salt

The optimal diet in the beginning would be to juice all fresh green foods and to have some freshly juiced wheat grass daily. You may have to start with one ounce a day and increase it from there. Wheat grass is very beneficial because it oxygenates the body and we've already discussed that cancer cannot survive in oxygen. So suck down all the oxygen you can get.

After reading this you're probably saying, "I can't survive on seeds and grass!" But don't worry. I have added some recipes that follow to get you started. It's not that bad, and as you feel better and your natural energy returns, you will be very happy that you've changed your diet.

WATER – IMPORTANCE OF GOOD ALKALINE WATER

In 1931 Dr. Otto Warburg was awarded the Nobel Prize for discovering the cause of cancer: "Cancer has one prime cause... and that is the replacement of oxygen (aerobic) respiration of body cells by anaerobic cell respiration." Cancer is a dark thing living in an acidic place devoid of oxygen. Alkaline Water penetrates body tissues bringing life-giving oxygen and minerals. Cancer is destroyed by oxygen. Early this century, at least one doctor cured his patients of cancer by giving them potash (potassium). Modern research indicates pre-cancerous cells do not become cancerous in the presence of calcium. Alkaline mineral salts neutralize poisonous acids while releasing oxygen as part of the reaction. Alkaline Water carries a **negative electrical charge** making it a natural antioxidant, and this electrical charge destroys bacteria, viruses and fungi. However, the electrical charge tends to disappear into the environment, so Alkaline Water cannot be stored for an extended time. It is best when fresh. Acid beverages such as soft drinks rob our bodies of oxygen, while alkaline drinks such as Alkaline Water enrich the body with oxygen and much needed minerals. Alkaline Water also neutralizes free radicals. There are several companies that sell these systems which range from $1500 to $5000. They are all great products; you be the judge on which one is best for you!"

Awareness is the first step to
healing and changing.
~ Louise L. Hay

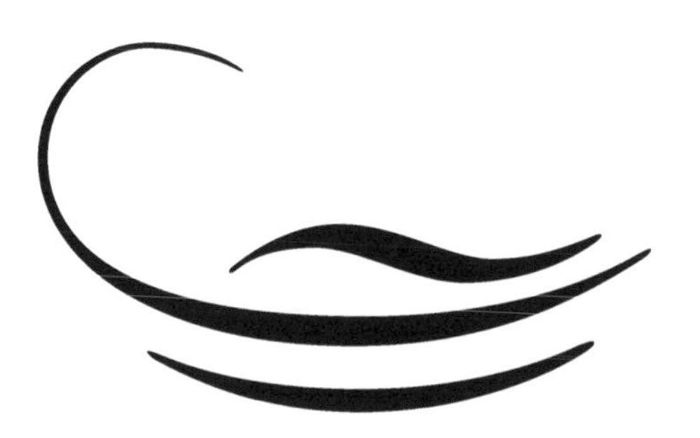

Chapter 12
Vitamin Suggestions

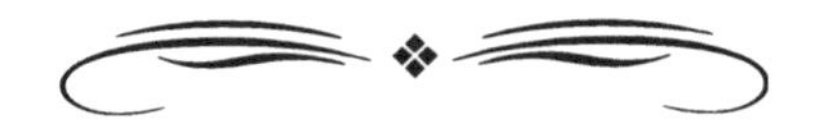

I WOULD SUGGEST THE FOLLOWING TO BE implemented immediately while reading the entire book. I feel very strongly about the Essiac Tea, and Coffee Enemas are a MUST!

Blend one organic lemon (including the pulp, peel the lemon) and drink with 8 oz. of water. Even though a lemon is a citrus fruit, it has an alkalizing effect on the body.

Essiac Tea for more information go to www.herbalhealer.com Herbal Healer Academy. Ask for their 4-Herb Tea. If you have breast cancer, consider adding red clover blossoms and

Montana yew tips to the brew. Perhaps other cancers respond to the last two ingredients also. Essiac Tea detoxifies the body and enhances the immune system.

Super Curcumin (800-544-4440) is a powerful, natural cancer fighting substance and it enhances the immune system. Curcumin acts as an antioxidant, destroys abnormal cells that can become cancerous, stops cancer cells from multiplying and blocks estrogen-mimicking chemicals that promote estrogen sensitive (breast and ovarian) cancer growth.

Co-enzyme Q10 - Q-Gel is the most potent and bio-available brand.

New research from Germany and the USA about a **Pineapple Cocktail**. US Nutritionist Dr. Norman Walker until the age of 116 believed that his secret to a healthy long life was vitamins in liquid. His tip for free Radicals is: Pineapple for pure enzymes. It supports your immune system and kills cancer cells as well as tumors.
Recipe: 3 rings of pineapple-fresh purified with one cup of buttermilk (or cottage cheese or Kefir) 3x per week.

Super Drink – Served in German clinics for cancer and the immune system.

Grind 2 tablespoons of flax seeds (use a coffee grinder) or use 1 tablespoon of organic cold pressed flaxseed oil, ½ cup organic yogurt or ½ cup organic cottage cheese and 1 cup organic Concord grape juice. Blend and drink. It's a great breakfast drink!

Protandim consisting of five synergistic herbs, activates Nrf2, a protein that regulates 500 of the 25,000 genes in the body that are termed survival genes. Survival genes come in three categories: antioxidant enzymes, anti-inflammatory genes, and anti-fibrotic genes (reduce scar tissue). One antioxidant gene was co-discovered by Dr. Joe McCord in 1969, SOD (Superoxide Dimutase) who formulated Protandim's five herbs: Tumeric, Green Tea, Milk Thistle, Ashwagandha Root, and Bacopa from hundreds tested. Protandim causes the body to turn up its ability to heal through its genome to create its own antioxidants and healing processes far more efficiently than simply ingesting other supplements. For additional information go to www.lifevantage.com/willbronson

ENZYMES - Wobenzym-N For inflammation, detoxification, and infection. Systemic enzymes have been found to be effective in the treatment of inflammation and infection due to bacteria, fungus, yeast, or virus. It is also very useful in treating joint disorders, cardio-vascular problems and traumatic injury. It has a high potency combination of pancreatin, bromelain, papain, rutin, trypsin. Go to www.modernherbalist.com for further information.

JUSURU LIFE BLEND – a cutting-edge liquid nutraceutical that contains the only liquid form of patented BioCell Collagen II in a matrix of joint and skin supporting hyaluronic acid, collagen, and chondroitin sulfate, in combination with exotic antioxidant-rich fruits from around the globe including mangosteen, acai berry, pomegranate, blueberry, goji, jujube and more. Jusuru also contains the equivalent amount of Resveratrol as two bottles of red wine in just a one ounce serving. Here are some of the key benefits of this product: It replenishes the levels of hyaluronic acid and collagen in your body by 60-fold. It helps to further prevent the breakdown of hyaluronic acid, as evident in a bioassay. Several double-blind, placebo-clinical trials have shown that BioCell Collagen II works by rebuilding your joint cartilage by feeding your body a naturally-occurring, all-natural, matrix of bioavailable collagen type II, hyaluronic acid, and chondroitin sulfate. Results of the studies showed significant improvement on joint health, mobility, stiffness, and all measures of the WOMAC scale. JUSURU is loaded with RESVERATROL. Resveratrol is a phytoalexin found in the skin of red grapes and is a constituent of red wine. It is a potent antioxidant that can activate a specific set of genes that scientists believe triggers life-extending survival mechanisms in the body. Call Ursula for additional information or visit the website at www.Jusuru.com/Ursula.

German Ozone recommended by Holistic Doctors is a therapy that removes your blood, oxygenates it, and is then replaced back into your body. Cancer cannot survive in an oxygenated environment.

Chealation as per Holistic Doctor – Vitamin Drips.

AMAS Testing - After a cancer diagnosis, take an AMAS test to see if you need more treatment. Or take the test to monitor your progress after treatment. (800-922-8378). AMAS test can detect cancer up to 18 months before any other test and is **FDA APPROVED**. Call for your free kit. It detects cancer in an undiagnosed person up to 19 months before doctor's test can pick it up. In a cancer patient, it allows a person to monitor the cancer activity in his body.

It's known as the 'French Paradox'... the mystery of how the French can smoke cigarettes, drink wine, and eat high-fat foods, while still having optimal health.

Meanwhile researchers call the potent polyphenols in Resveratrol found in red wine an anti-aging wonder... a proverbial 'fountain of youth'...* But the alcohol, sugar, and calories in wine can negatively impact your health and wreck your insulin levels, so I don't recommend getting your Resveratrol that way.

A water soluble antioxidant, **Purple Defense** helps you neutralize free radicals. It crosses the blood-brain barrier to help protect your brain and nervous system, and help support your immune system which may increase your cells' lifespan - and help provide energy and vitality.*

Its lipid soluble cousin, **Astaxanthin**, is a super-carotenoid more powerful than beta carotene and vitamins A, and E. It helps reduce wrinkles, dry skin, and age spots... and helps protect your eyes and brain from oxidative stress.

Additional Research found on the internet in regard to Resveratrol:

Scholarly articles for Resveratrol Cancer Research
http://www.google.com/search?q=resveratrol+cancer+research&rlz=1I7ACAW_enUS369&ie=UTF-8&oe=UTF-8&sourceid=ie7

Resveratrol inhibits the expression and function of the ... - Mitchell - Cited by 154
http://cancerres.aacrjournals.org/content/59/23/5892.short

Cancer chemo preventative activity of Resveratrol, a ... - Jang - Cited by 2539
http://www.chiroonline.net/_fileCabinet/scienceresveratrol.pdf

Resveratrol induces growth inhibition, S-phase arrest, ... - Joe - Cited by 223
http://www.erbeofficinali.org/dati/nacci/studi/Resveratrolo%20induce%20APOPTOSI%20su%20vari%20tipi%20di%20cancro.pdf

It is important to see a Chiropractor in your neighborhood. "It is most necessary to know the nature of the spine. One or more vertebrae may or may not go out of place very much and if they do, they are likely to produce serious complications. If not properly adjusted. Many diseases are related to the spine" The nervous system controls and coordinates all of the organs and structures of the human body. The spine is the lifeline. www.mynapleschiropractor.com

Acupuncture is also a must and why: The acupuncturist is able to influence health and sickness by stimulating certain areas along these "meridians". Traditionally these areas or "acupoints" were stimulated by fine, slender needles. Today, many additional forms of stimulation are incorporated, including herbs, electricity, magnets and lasers. Still, the aim remains the same - adjust the "vital energy" so the proper amount reaches the proper place at the proper time. This helps your body heal itself.

- **Lymphatic System**
- Proper Hydration
- Exercise and Body Movement
- Rebounding (bouncing up and down on mini trampoline)
- 85 % of the immune system is contained within the lymph. The lymph is a separate sewage system / drain for waste.
- Skin Brushing, see details in detox section
- **Baking Soda** – Skin Cancer – make with water and paste and put it on the area over night. In an aluminum free baking soda *BOB'S RED MILL* brand 1- 2 teaspoons in water is a power alkalizer (1–2 times a day) ADD TO ALKALINE WATER

The Need To Detox your Emotions!

Words have the power to both destroy and heal. When words are both true and kind, they can change our world.

~ Louise L. Hay

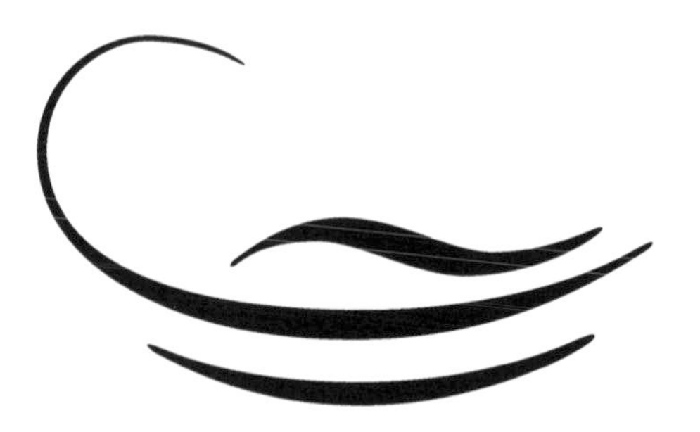

Chapter 13

Ursula's Meal Plan and Favorite Recipes

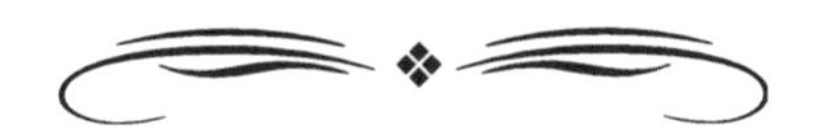

I SHOP AT MY LOCAL FARMERS MARKET ON Saturday for the whole week in Naples. We are lucky to have three farmers with organic fruits and vegetables. It is very hard for me to follow a recipe, so I just mix my own ingredients and whatever I have in my refrigerator. You can do the same and just substitute different vegetables for the day or the week.

BREAKFAST AND LUNCH

Steal cut OAT MEAL - Organic oat meal cooked in good water, sweetened by a bit of honey, banana, prune (soak overnight)

SMOOTHIE - I make my own Kefir very day. Combine the kefir with ¼ piece of pineapple, one banana, pinch of turmeric, maybe some orange juice and 4 tablespoons of hemp.

Mix it in a blender and this is my smoothie.

Juicing: To enhance taste I add an apple, ginger and lemon to my different juices. Ingredients- 1 apple or 1 pear, 1 lemon, some ginger, and any combination of kale, cabbage, spinach or cucumbers, tomatoes, dandelion, peppers, celery, small portion of arugula, carrots, 4-5 asparagus. More asparagus than that is too bitter. (Beets for different flavor, I love the greens from the beets, zucchini, broccoli, cauliflower.) **Anything that is green I buy at the farmers market.**

At the end of the week, all veggies left over are put into my Vita-Mix with warm water and vegetable bouillon to make stock for future soups. I will freeze the ingredients in a glass container. If it is too green and bitter, I might be lazy and add a can of organic soup (Amy's Lentil Vegetable or Wolfgang Puck's Organic Tomato Basil Bisque.)

You may also add a tomato, carrots, or sweat potatoes for flavor.

LUNCH

SALADS - I love kale chopped very small in my salad with beans, parsnip fresh from the market, cucumbers, small portions of arugula, cilantro and fresh basil with other fresh herbs to enhance the salad. I also will add in Goat Cheese or Feta Cheese too. I make my own salad dressing using lemon juice, good oil, a touch balsamic vinegar, fresh herbs. Excellent.

SOUP – Chop up 3 med. carrots, 1 large parsnip, 1 large potato, 1 onion, ¼ cup water with ½ cup of vegetable broth. Cook.

SNACKS - Apples, Nuts (Brazilian and Almonds soaked)

HUMMUS - 15 oz. (one can of organic chick peas drained,) ½ cup raw sesame seeds, 1 tablespoon olive oil, ¼ cup lemon juice, 1 clove of garlic, and roasted tomatoes and/or peppers. Put in blender. One of my favorite snacks.

DINNER

SOUPS - One hand full of spinach, 4 large carrots, ½ pepper, 1 stem of kale, 2 med. tomatoes, ½ sweet potato, 1 stem celery, ½ cup beans or lentils (optional), Fresh ginger, fresh basil, fresh cilantro - Mix in blender. **Add** 1 cup boiled water with 1 cube of vegetable bouillon.

SALAD with Vegan burgers or salmon for additional protein.

SALT - Your salt should be mined in the Himalayas – GO TO www.PowerOrganics.com. It has a great taste and will enhance the natural flavor of your food with 72 different minerals.

During my cancer fight I was very strict for one year and now call myself a cheating vegan. I mostly, out of consciousness, do not eat meat, chicken, or turkey. I do make exceptions with fish. At home I make homemade kefir which is a yogurt substitute and very healthy. On vacation I eat almost everything except meat and poultry.

CHARLES' FAVORITE RECIPES
For Health & Wellness

SWEET POTATO SOUP *Ingredients*	
1 cup water with 1 tablespoon nutritional yeast or soup stock	
3 cups sweet potato	1 cup parsnip (optional)
½ cup fresh parsley	¼ cup onion
Organic fermented soy sauce to taste	1 teaspoon dill
1 cup fresh carrot juice	Sea salt to taste
Preparation - Grate sweet potato, parsnip, chop onion and mince parsley. Place remainder of the vegetables in bowls and cover with soup.	

NRG SOUP *Ingredients*	
Soup Base	**Other Ingredients cont.**
2 cucumbers, peeled	½ Cup fresh corn
½ Cup lemon juice	1 tablespoon minced garlic
½ tomato	½ tablespoon minced ginger
Other Ingredients	½ Tablespoon hot pepper chopped
1 cup diced tomato	1/3 Cup Tamari or Nama Shoyu
1 cup chopped mint	1 Medium apple. Chopped
½ Cup chopped onion	2 Cups orange juice_
½ Cup red pepper	

Preparation - Soup base: In a blender, blend cucumbers, lemon, and tomato until smooth.

Place "soup base" into blender and add remaining ingredients and blend until smooth. Garnish with mung bean sprouts, diced peppers, green onions, or chopped sea weed.

If you want your soup to be more like a chunky gaspacho style soup then blend the soup base and add the finely diced vegetable stock without blending a second time. This way you have a soup stock and some vegetables you can chew.

THE SEED CHEESE *Ingredients*	
¼ cup fresh lemon juice	¼ red bell pepper
¼ cup Nama Shoyu	2-3 cloves garlic, peeled
1-1 ½ cups raw cashews, macadamia nuts, pine nuts, or a combination	
Preparation - In a high speed blender, combine all of the filling ingredients and blend until the resulting cashew cheese in uniform and smooth.	

CREAMY TOMATO BASIL SOUP *Ingredients*	
1 ½ cups thai coconut water	3 cups blended tomato 4-5 medium tomato
1 stalk celery	¼ cup lemon juice
¼ yellow onion	¼ cup olive oil
1 cup fresh basil	¼ cup Tamari
5 cloves garlic	1 teaspoon sea salt
Preparation - Combine ingredients and blend until smooth - Garnish with fresh cilantro, dill, mint, oregano, or tarragon	

THAI NOODLES WITH MOCK PEANUT SAUCE *Ingredients*	
2 large zucchini	**Mock peanut sauce:**
1 ½ tablespoons Minced fresh chives	½ cup sesame oil
1 tablespoon sesame oil	¼ cup date paste
1 ½ teaspoons tamari sauce	2 tablespoons fine chopped ginger
½ teaspoon sea salt	2 tablespoons light miso
Pinch cayenne	1 teaspoon sea salt
1 ½ tablespoons sesame seeds	1 tablespoon raw apple cider vinegar
1 tablespoon minced lemon grass	

Preparation -
Thai noodles: Grate zucchini in a spirilizer to make thin angel hair style noodles. Then combine remaining ingredients in bowl and mix with the noodles.

Mock peanut sauce: Combine ingredients in blender and blend until smooth. Place sauce in side bowl with noodles or serve on top of noodles.

RAW CHILI *Ingredients*	
1 Teaspoon of Garlic	2 Teaspoons of Basil
2 Tablespoons of Cumin	2 Tablespoons of nutritional Yeast
1 Teaspoon of Oregano	2 Tablespoons of fermented soy sauce
6 Cup of Tomatoes	½ Cup of corn Kernels
1 Cup of Onion	1 cup of red pepper
1 Clove of Garlic	1 cup of bulgar wheat
3 stocks of celery	

Preparation - Juice tomatoes to equal 3 cups of juice; Squeeze lemon, mince garlic; finely chop onion, bell peppers and celery. Chop 3 cup of tomatoes, and remove corn kernels, place in bowl and allow flavors to mingle.

Serve chilled or slightly warmed.

RAW VEGETARIAN LASAGNA WITH BASIL-PISTACHIO PESTO AND PIGNOLI RICOTTA

Ingredients

Pignoli ricotta:	1 tablespoons sea salt
2 cups raw pignoli nuts, soaked 1 hr minimum	6 tablespoons clean water
2 tablespoons lemon juice	
Place pignoli nuts, lemon juice, nutritional yeast, and sea salt into food processor and pulse few minutes until thoroughly combines. Gradually add the water and process until the texture becomes fluffy like ricotta. Then set aside.	
Basil-pistachio pesto:	¼ cup plus 2 tablespoons extra virgin olive oil
2 cups packed basil leaves	1 teaspoon sea salt
½ cup pistachios soaked 1 hour min	Pinch black pepper
Place the pesto ingredients into a food processor and blend until well combined but still chunky. Set aside.	
Tomato sauce;	6 medium tomatoes
½ cup yellow onion chopped	*Continues*

Raw Vegetarian Lasagna with Basil-Pistachio Pesto and Pignoli Ricotta Continued *Ingredients*	
4 tablespoons extra virgin olive oil	Pinch black pepper
2 teaspoons sea salt	2 teaspoons Italian seasoning
2 tablespoons raw agave nectar	
Cover food dehydrator tray with parchment paper and smother with olive oil. Slice tomatoes into ½ thick pieces and place onto tray (usually 3 tomatoes to each tray). Sprinkle spices, slat, and agave onto tomatoes and dehydrate at 105 degrees for 4-5 hours until tomatoes are 30-50% Reduced. Then smash them together into pasty consistency. Set aside	
Cut three zucchini into thin strips lengthwise, (very thin pieces) then place into mixing bowl with 2 tablespoons olive oil and Italian spices, pinch sea salt. When coverd layer zucchini onto pan and cover layer with ricotta, tomato sauce, basil-pistachio pesto, and then thin slice tomato. Make three layers and decorate top with small diced red and yellow peppers. May place into food dehydrator or short time to warm slightly	

SEA VEGETABLE SALAD *Ingredients*	
For the pickled cherries:	***For the Salad:***
1 cup sour cherries, pitted and halved	1 ounce dried wakame
½ cup vinegar, preferably apple cider vinegar	1 ounce dried hijiki
3 tablespoons agave nectar	1 ounce dried arame
For the sweet Miso Dressing:	1 large cucumber, peeled, seeded, and julienned
½ cup white miso	2 large beets, peeled and julienned
1/3 cup agave nectar	1 medium dakion radish, peeled and julienned
¼ cup soy sauce	2 tablespoons black sesame seeds
¼ cup sesame oil	2 tablespoons white sesame seeds
¼ cup lemon juice	½ sheet dry nori
¼ cup chopped ginger	1 green onion, white and 1 inch of green very thinly sliced
	continues...

SEA VEGETABLE SALAD... *continued*

Preparation - In separate bowls, soak the sea vegetables in water until soft. Wait five to ten minutes to drain off the water. The hijiki and wakame may take up to 20 minutes. Drain the sea vegetables, using your hands, squeeze out as much of the water as possible. Roughly chop the wakame into smaller pieces. Place the sea vegetables in a large bowl and add the cucumber, beets, radish, and pickled cherries. Add about half of the dressing to the vegetables and toss gently to combine. Sprinkle with the green onion and both black and white sesame seeds.

<table>
<tr><td colspan="2">RAW SPAGHETTI
Ingredients: Marinara Sauce</td></tr>
<tr><td>1 ripe tomato, seeded and chopped (about ½ cup)</td><td>½ cup sun-dried tomatoes, soaked or oil-packed</td></tr>
<tr><td>½ red bell pepper, chopped (about ½ cup)</td><td>½ tsp plus 1/8 tsp salt</td></tr>
<tr><td>2 tbsp extra-virgin olive oil</td><td>Dash black pepper (optional)</td></tr>
<tr><td>1 tbsp minced fresh basil, or 1 tsp dried</td><td>Dash cayenne</td></tr>
<tr><td>1 tsp dried oregano</td><td></td></tr>
<tr><td colspan="2">Ingredients: Spaghetti</td></tr>
<tr><td colspan="2">Zucchini and/or yellow squash (approximately 1 per person)</td></tr>
<tr><td colspan="2"><u>Preparation</u> -
Marinara Sauce: Place all the ingredients in a food processor and process until smooth. Store in sealed container in the refrigerator. Marinara sauce will keep for 3 days.

Spaghetti: Using a Japanese vegetable grater, grate zucchini into "angel hair pasta". Strain juice, top with marinara sauce, and serve</td></tr>
</table>

<table>
<tr><td colspan="2">VEGETARIAN NORI ROLLS
Ingredients:</td></tr>
<tr><td>Nori sheets</td><td>1 cup sunflower sprouts</td></tr>
<tr><td>1 Red pepper (cut into thin strips)</td><td>1 avocado (Thin slices)</td></tr>
<tr><td>1 Yellow pepper (cut into thin strips)</td><td>1 green onion (Thin cut strips)</td></tr>
<tr><td colspan="2">Head of red leaf lettuce or Chinese cabbage (thin cut strips)</td></tr>
<tr><td colspan="2">1 cucumber thin slice and de seeded (dry moisture before using)</td></tr>
<tr><td>1 carrot cut into match stick sizes</td><td>Wasabi powder</td></tr>
<tr><td>May use sesame tahini paste</td><td>For dipping sauce may use fermented soy sauce</td></tr>
<tr><td colspan="2">Place nori sheets into dehydrator at 105 degrees to make crisper nori

Lay out sheet and place shredded greens and then place stripped vegetables lengthwise. Roll nori into tight roll. Use Moist wasab paste to seal the edge of nori roll when tightly rolled. Use sparingly as wasbi can have quite a kick in the sinus cavity if too much is used. Cut inot half and serve.</td></tr>
</table>

<table>
<tr><td colspan="2">FLAX SEED CRACKERS
Ingredients:</td></tr>
<tr><td>2 cups flax seeds, soak ½-2 hours</td><td>1 cup dried tomatoes, chopped</td></tr>
<tr><td>½ cup red pepper, chopped</td><td>1 tablespoon olive oil</td></tr>
<tr><td>¼ cup fresh cilantro, chopped</td><td>1 teaspoon sea salt</td></tr>
<tr><td colspan="2">(May add 1-2 teaspoons garlic powder, onion powder, Italian seasonings)</td></tr>
<tr><td colspan="2">Mix all ingredients with the flax seeds</td></tr>
<tr><td colspan="2">Spread mixture into desired shape. Score for even cutting. Dehydrate at 105 degrees for about 5 hours or until desired crispness

Turn over after 2-3 hours for even drying.</td></tr>
</table>

FOR ADDITIONAL RECIPES FROM CHARLES GO TO www.AskCharlesMarble.com

When you take excellent care
of yourself, everybody benefits.
Give yourself a relaxing treat
today, such as a massage,
sea salt bath, or pedicure.
~ Louise L. Hay

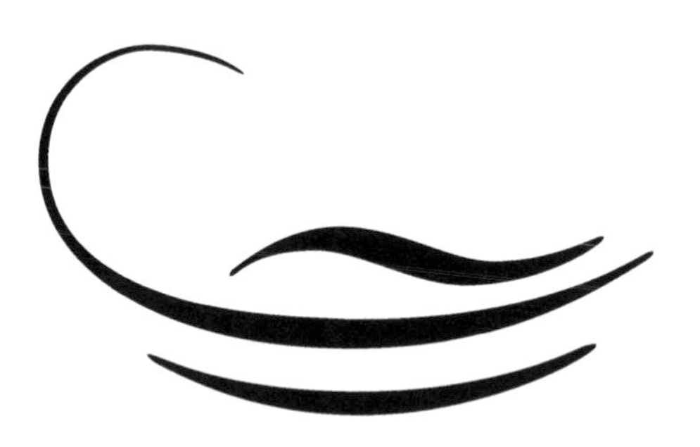

Chapter 14

How to Detoxify The Body!

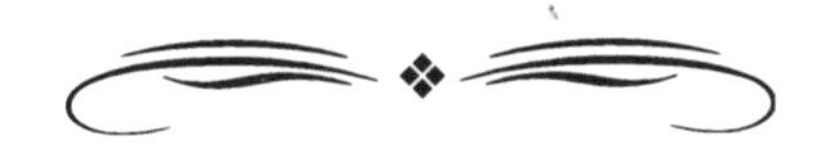

NOW THAT WE KNOW BETTER AND are not loading our body up with toxins anymore (and this means, toxic foods, toxic environment, toxic emotions) we also have to eliminate the toxins that we've been putting in there for years. This is what separates the men from the boys. This is where you really have to get down to it and WANT to survive. Detoxifying can be done on many levels of intensity, and the protocols that outlined here are for maximum detoxification in a minimal amount of time. Please work with a health care provider. It is very important that you have someone monitoring your healing process. Oftentimes during detoxifying we go through what is known as a "healing crisis." This is where the toxins are holding on to us for dear life, (it's them or you) and your body is giving it everything it's got to push them out. Some examples of "healing crisis" symptoms are diarrhea, sweating, fainting, shaking, headaches, etc. for maybe 3-5 days.

The Detoxification Process

Along with changing your diet, you must **CLEANSE** your internal body systems to start the healing process. It is also highly recommended to continue these principals throughout your lifetime. Consider doing a complete body cleanse program every other month for at the first year, then at least four times per year.

Internal cleansing is a foundation in health. Internal cleansing has been understood for hundreds of years in natural cancer therapies. The emphasis is based on helping the body eliminate its waste; this in turn reduces blockages that restrict optimum health. There are hundreds of different ways to cleanse the body naturally. Some are more expensive, drastic and detailed then others. Some are fairly cheap, easy and efficient. Depending on your specific body type there are many ways to personalize the perfect cleanse for you. What is most important is choosing the right plan for you and sticking to it! Diligence is what pays the dividends. Consistency is what yields the greatest results.

The principle areas to begin cleansing are the organ systems associated with elimination. The key organs to focus on are the colon, liver, kidneys, lymphatic system, and the skin. Keeping these systems open and properly functioning is vital.

Coffee Enemas

A lifetime of living on a so called normal diet can block the liver. As you start to eat and drink the nutrient rich foods, the cells are rapidly absorbing and forcing toxins from the cells into the bloodstream, which in turn transports them to the liver, the body's chief organ of detoxification. As a result the liver may be unable to deal with the newly arriving toxins driven from the tissues by live nutrients. Unless quickly shifted, this log jam of toxins could lead to threatening self intoxication and liver coma, hence the vital role of rapidly detoxifying with coffee enemas. There are many methods of cancer therapies that can kill tumor tissue, but it is vital to remove the dead toxic material from the liver. Dr Max Gerson's use of coffee enemas to detoxify the liver was confirmed by three scientists from the Department of Pathology, University of Minnesota. The tests proved that rectal coffee administration stimulates an enzyme system in the liver, which is able to remove toxic free radicals from the bloodstream. The normal activity of this enzyme is increased by 600-700 % by the coffee enemas. This greatly increases detoxification, is rich in potassium, and helps prevent intestinal cramping. A recent 1990 study of six years with a group of 60 cancer patients had amazing results, including reduction in all pain medications, slowing liver metastases, and even complete remission without conventional therapy.

Coffee Enema Instructions

For 1 Coffee Enema:

3 large rounded tablespoons of organic ground coffee in 2 cups boiling water. Bring to slow boil, remove from heat and let stand 15 minuets. Drain coffee grounds and you are left with a coffee concentrate.

Place coffee concentrate in enema bucket or enema bag and filled with distilled water to equal a total of 32 ounces. Lay on your right side and slowly add coffee into rectum. If an urge to expel occurs, stop and wait until urge diminishes. Continue filling colon. If you must expel, stop, expel and then continue filling with remaining coffee liquid. Lay in fetal position for 15 min on right side. After 5 minutes slowly sit up and expel.

For 3 Coffee Enemas:

Use 1 quart of distilled water and bring to a boil, add 9 tablespoons organic coffee, boil 2 minutes, reduce heat and let stand 15 minutes. Drain and portion out coffee concentrate between 3 coffee enemas.

Store unused coffee in refrigerator until needed.

Basic Colon Cleanse

The first place to start in internal cleansing is the colon. There is an old adage, "all disease starts in the intestine." It's a good reminder to start with the intestines.

In order to cleanse the colon, you must change your diet. The necessary foods are high in soluble fiber, which helps to lubricate the intestinal wall, made in elimination of waste more efficient. Bitter foods are better for the liver. After simply tasting bitter foods on your tongue, you immediately stimulate bile flow from the liver. Bile plays an important role in stimulating peristalsis in the intestine. Peristalsis is the wave like muscular activity that moves our waste through our intestine. Adding bitter foods in the diet not only helps cleanse the liver, but also the intestine. Historically humans originally included bitter foods in their diet. Throughout the years we have replaced this key component with sweet and salty foods.

Another factor is proper hydration. Proper hydration lubricates the intestinal walls which aids the elimination of waste. We receive hydration through water and fresh foods that are high in water content. Fresh fruits and vegetables are loaded with both water and soluble fiber.

Foods that lubricate the intestine and stimulate bile flow:

· Aloe Vera
· Chia Seeds
· Bananas
· Almonds
· Sweet Potato
· Peaches
· Pears
· Plums
· Prunes
· Apricots
· Spinach
· All dark green leafy vegetables and bitter foods

COLON Cleansing

Just a reminder to hear again "all disease starts in the intestine" so start with the intestines. Use the foods that treat constipation.

- Consider using an herbal colon cleanse product of choice. There are many various forms on the market, many containing the same base ingredients.

- A few examples are Renu Life Cleanse Smart, Turkey Rhubarb capsules. Dr. Schulze intestinal formula.

- Pick a product and take as directed. Increase your daily dosage until bowels move 2-3 times daily. Stool should be soft and not too loose. If too loose back off your dosage until good daily bowel habits are established.

- After one week of starting the colon cleanse formula it can be helpful to use a bulking formula to scrub the inside walls of the intestine.

- A good standing product is Dr. Schulze intestinal 2 formula. There are many comparable forms to this brand. Most contain activated charcoal, psyllium, bentonite clay, flax seed powder, slippery elm powder, marshmallow root powder. Use as directed 1 teaspoon in 4-8 ounces of water 6 times daily for 10 days.

- Another incredible and low cost way to clean the colon is to use peroxide enemas.
  · Use 35% food grade peroxide only (see sources)
  · Use 50 drops of food grade peroxide to 32 ounces of water in enema bag. Each day increase by 5 drops until you reach 100 drops. When reaching 100 drops maintain at 100 drops each time. The food grade

peroxide is oxygen and water, nothing else. It helps to scrub the inside intestinal walls with oxygen as a "scrub brush" many if not most all who have used the peroxide enemas have been astounded by the waste, parasites, yeast, and worms that are removed. For true effects, you might consider increasing to twice daily for at least 4 weeks or longer.

- Coffee enemas have been around in cancer therapies for over 100 years. Has been argued by some that coffee is too acidic and stimulating for the body.
  · Even though the counter arguments exist and sound good in theory. Coffee enemas have been and still are foundations for many alternative cancer physicians around the world.

- Dr. Max Gerson would recommend up to four coffee enemas each day, and would even go so far to tell his cancer patients not to drink his 13 glasses of carrot juice daily unless they did the coffee enemas. The coffee when instilled into the large intestine is moved by the portal vein system directly to the liver, which causes the liver to purge its waste and bile.

- If using coffee enemas be sure to use the strongest organic fresh ground coffee. Conventional coffee beans are one of the most sprayed imports we have and are known to contain harmful chemical compounds. It is best to make your coffee and let stand until room temperature before using in enema. A good technique when doing the coffee enema is to use half the enema bag, and release it, then instill the remaining 1/2 and hold as long as tolerated before releasing to get the best effect.

Now Is The Perfect Time to Flush the Liver!

A basic cheap liver flush - First thing in the morning:

- One clove garlic
- One tablespoon olive oil
- 8 ounces citrus juice
- Quarter cup fresh parsley
- Blend together drink

Increase by one on the olive oil and garlic to suite your tolerance, 5 would be the max.
Wait a half hour to an hour and drink 2 cups of a detox tea.

- 8-10 apricots in the blender with water drink that and then eat the pits.

That compliments the bile flow, lubricates and hydrates the intestine.

- The following is prepartion for a stronger liver flush, and do for 2 days:

- 32 ounces in apple juice or citrus juice (8 lemons) to pre-soften bile / gal stones.

- 3rd day- half teaspoon of Epsom salts in four ounces of water exactly at 6 pm.

- Repeat at 8 pm
  · Epsom salts are Magnesium which dilates the common bile duct and allows for stone and bile to flow.

- 10 pm take one cup of olive oil, the juice of one grape fruit shake and drink quickly.
  · Immediately lie in bed, curl your legs up in fetal position
  · If nauseous chew on a little bit of ginger to settle the stomach.

- Following morning 8 am Epsom salts and water

- 10 am repeat

- Compliment that with a couple cups of detox tea

Look for small pea size to golf ball sized stones. Another thing to compliment liver cleansing is hot castor oil packs over the liver to help open the liver and flush.

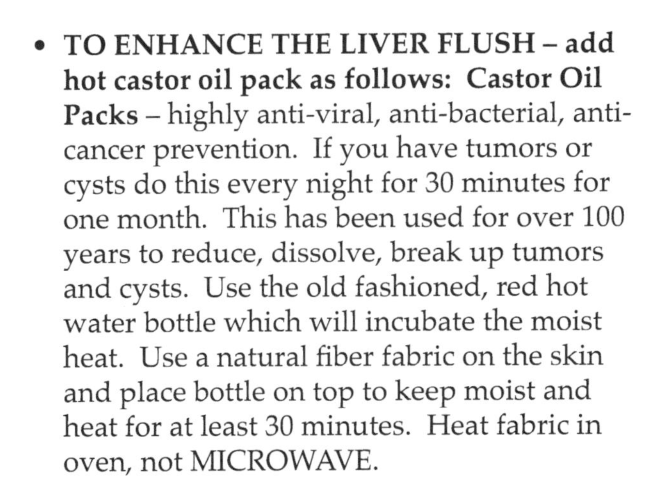

- **TO ENHANCE THE LIVER FLUSH – add hot castor oil pack as follows: Castor Oil Packs** – highly anti-viral, anti-bacterial, anti-cancer prevention. If you have tumors or cysts do this every night for 30 minutes for one month. This has been used for over 100 years to reduce, dissolve, break up tumors and cysts. Use the old fashioned, red hot water bottle which will incubate the moist heat. Use a natural fiber fabric on the skin and place bottle on top to keep moist and heat for at least 30 minutes. Heat fabric in oven, not MICROWAVE.

After cleaning the Liver it is good to Flush the Kidneys!

Simple Kidney Flush Suggestions:

- Use one bag of a kidney tea of which there are many variations. A good tea for the kidneys will often contain juniper berries, gravel root, hydrangea, corn silk, uva ursi, marshmallow root, dandelion root, pipsesewa.

- Use about 4-6 ounces of dry herbs and place into 96 ounces of apple juice, the juice of 10 lemons or limes, 10 ounces of raw apple cider vinegar. Let mixture stand on your counter over night. The next day strain and drink 4 ounces on the hour every hour for two days.

- Detox teas are very helpful and aid the liver, kidneys, lymph and colon.

- It is helpful to alternate your teas every month or two. When consuming herbs and even the same foods over long periods of time, it is a good idea to alternate your foods or herbs. The longer we take the same foods or herbs each day, the more the body becomes sensitized by them. Historically we had changes of season which forced us to alter our diets. Now we have the "convenience" of having the same food sources available to use each and every day.

- Well established detox tea examples to alternate every few months are:

- Essiac tea 4-8 ounces daily

- Jason winters tea 8-32 ounces daily

- Dr. Schulze detox tea 32 ounces daily.

- Hilda Clarks herbal detox tea recipe 32 ounces daily

- When making the teas be sure to use pure water, and make in a glass or stainless steal pot. Boil as directed and steep over night before straining. The longer steeping times will help to increase the potency of the teas.

Sweat therapy or hyperthermia is also a long standing therapy dating back to Hypocrites'.

- The systemic heat induction opens the circulation, moves the lymph, and the sweating helps the body eliminate waste. Every degree of temperature increase in the body doubles the speed activity of your white blood cells. Also cancer cells have demonstrated an inability to tolerate temperatures above 101 degrees.
- Steam saunas, Far infrared saunas, zone steam saunas are all great ways to eliminate waste, increase immune response, and provide a hostile environment for cancer cells.
- On a sunny summer day, one can often just roll up the windows of their car and park directly into the sun and in just a few minutes you have a sauna.
- Hot Epsom salt and baking soda baths are also a good way to compliment the hyperthermia. It is best to have a water filtration system in place before using the hot bath therapies as common municipal water sources are high in chlorine and a wide arrange of other harmful chemicals. You can absorb a pond of water weight within one hour of soaking in water, so be sure the water is clean before using bath therapies.

- Simple low cost recipe—2 to 4 cups Epsom salts and 1 cup baking soda. The Epsom salts are all magnesium and sodium which makes an isotonic solution that helps to draw waste from the body. The baking soda is an alkaline neutralizer and has even demonstrated to be helpful in reducing radiations harmful effects on the body. If using the bath therapies, be sure to get the water as hot as tolerated and soak at least 30 minutes.
- Another old fashioned hyperthermia bath treatment is the cold sheet treatment. It's very powerful and not for the faint of heart.
- Fill bath tub with water as hot as you can possible tolerate. Grind at least 2 bulbs of fresh garlic, about 4 inches of fresh ginger, 1/2 cup of fresh ground mustard seeds, and a handful of fresh hot pepper of choice or 1/2 cup of cayenne powder. Place herbs into a woman's stocking or sock. Tie the end off to prevent herbs from washing out and plugging drain. Squeeze the herbal combination into the bath water and leave herbs to soak in water.
- Coat your genitals and rectum with castor oil, or un-petroleum jelly (sold in health food stores) this will prevent discomfort from the heat of the herbs when soaking.
- Place a 100% cotton sheet into ice water and let soak.

- Sit in hot bath and soak as deep as you can in the tube while drinking six cups of yarrow tea (see sources) within 30 minutes.

- Then get out of bath and have person wring out cotton sheet and wrap around body covering as much skin area as possible. Then go directly to bed and cover with warm blankets to incubate the heart and stay in sheet in bed as long as tolerated, over night is best.

- In the old days the feet were rubbed in bed with petroleum jelly and packed with ground garlic and ground mustard seeds to increase the detoxification. They also use to do a garlic enema before doing the bath, all of which can be used to increase the effectiveness of the bath treatment.

- This is one of the most powerful herbal treatments ever known. It also seems to get easier after the first time. If tolerated would be good to use once week while detoxifying.

- When doing this treatment it is good to have someone there to assist you and comfort you.

- A much easier form of hydro therapy that should be included is hot and cold showers. Be sure to have at least a shower filter on your shower before using shower treatments. In any event, one should at least have a shower filter to reduce the amounts of harmful chemicals. Alternate the water temp as hot as you can tolerate for 2-3 minutes and then turn the hot water off and use cold water for 2-3 minutes. Alternate back and forth as long as tolerated each day to help move lymph flow. Hand held shower attachments are great to use since they allow focusing directly to areas of concern. The hot water increases the circulation and the cold water restricts the circulation.

- Fasting is also another long established way to help the body detoxify. Juice fasting is common, meaning only drinking juices and no solid foods for 3-4 weeks.
- The master cleanse is a water style fast that is in many ways better than just using water.
- **Lymphatic System**
- Proper Hydration
- Exercise and Body Movement
- Rebounding (bouncing up and down on mini trampoline)

85 % of the immune system is contained within the lymph. The lymph is a separate sewage system / drain for waste.

- Skin Brushing

Detox Skin Brushing: A Swift and Powerful Home Detox

Our skin is the largest elimination organ and responsible for 10% to 15% of body elimination. Dry skin brushing is an easy, quick, and powerful way to enhance your detoxification with tremendous benefits! Why? It stimulates blood circulation, is a lymphatic cleanser, enhances toxin elimination while improving the over appearance of your skin. Skin brushing will eliminate dead cells and assists in regenerating our skin.

Our lymphatic system is composed of lymph vessels, lymph nodes, and organs which is part of the body's defense system. Lymph nodes remove microorganisms and other foreign substances which act as a filtration system that keeps particulate matter, example - bacteria, from entering the bloodstream.

All that is needed for skin brushing is a NATURAL bristle brush with a long handle or a loofah and only 5 minutes. Brush the skin when it is dry and follow with a hot shower to wash off the dead cells. Begin with brushing your feet, including the soles, moving upwards toward the heart, in small circular motions. For upper body put one arm up and brush downward towards your armpit and the same process on the other side. You will brush down towards the heart. Concentrate on the breast and armpit areas where there's a concentration of lymph nodes. Brush the abdominal area from left to right using the circle motion to gently massage the colon. Spending time on your thighs and hips is also excellent to work on the cellulite areas as well. Then complete the body by finishing off around the neck and shoulders.

As a guide, it is beneficial to brush from the extremities up or down to the core of the body.

How do you brush? Please brush gently especially over sensitive areas. Over time and practice, your skin will become more resilient and will endure more vigorous brushing. Avoid brushing over any cuts, irritated areas, or bruises.

The benefits of dry brushing are the following: accelerates elimination of toxicity, enhances lymphatic flow, stimulates circulation and blood flow, exfoliates and removes dead skin, it is anti-aging with cell regeneration, stimulates the sebaceous and sweat glands which enhances restoration of supple and moist skin, and reduces cellulite to name a few.

ICING ON THE CAKE...

I highly suggest you finish with a 10 minute cold detox bath which will be far superior to any detox spa treatment you will experience and it is **FREE!** The father of detoxification, Louis Kuhne of Leipzig from the 1880s, is proven to encourage toxin, waste and fat elimination. The detox bath's working principle is to refresh the core area of the body (groin) for 10 minutes daily. This process creates a vibration in the fascia (interconnecting tissue covering all internal organs), which sets in motion a roll-back effect transporting waste, fat and deposited toxins back to the intestines, where they are later eliminated.

What will you experience from skin brushing and the cold detox bath? A significant improvement in your toxin elimination, feel rejuvenated, and renewed energy.

Old Fashioned Castor Oil Remedy

- Need – castor oil, hot water bottle, organic unbleached natural wool towel (found in most health food stores).
- Pour castor oil onto wool pad and place into oven until hot to touch, but does not burn skin (no microwaves)
- Place wool pad over affected area on skin on castor oil side of pad touching skin.
- For best results use multiple layers of Castor oil pads, 4 layers saturated with Castor oil.
- Cover pads with hot water bottle which should stay hot for 2 hours.
- Do not use electric heating pads due to harmful effects of EMFs.

- The hot water bottle will incubate the heat and open the pores of the skin.
- To reduce messy effects of Castor oil packs, you can cover the Castor oil pad with saran wrap after applying to skin to keep oil from spreading around if desired).
- For best results be sure to keep Castor oil packs on affected area for 30 minutes or longer each day.

The Master Cleanse Recipe:

The Master Cleanse works just how it sounds; you consume primarily lemonade for the entire time you're on the diet. So the recipes for the diet itself are fairly simple. You should drink a minimum of 60 oz. of lemonade a day, but can drink more if you like. You can also drink as much water as you want. I suggest you consume your body weight in ounces of water.
Below are two different recipes. The first is for a single serving of the master cleanse lemonade. The second will make 6 servings

✓ **Single Serving:**

- 2 Tablespoons of organic lemon Juice (about 1/2 a Lemon)
- 2 Tablespoons of Organic grade B maple syrup (not the commercial maple flavored syrup you use on pancakes)

- 1/10 Teaspoon Cayenne pepper powder
- Ten ounces of filtered water

✓ **Six Servings – 60 oz:**

- 60 ounces of filtered water
- 12 Tablespoons of organic grade B maple syrup
- 12 Tablespoons of organic lemon juice
- 1/2 Teaspoon cayenne pepper powder
- There are a couple important things to remember when preparing the lemonade.
- For one, the lemon juice used must be fresh squeezed. This cannot be emphasized enough. It is necessary to use fresh produce. Canned juice won't work and will erase most of the benefits of using the master cleanser diet.
- Also, the maple syrup must be grade B maple syrup, not the sugar filled syrup that is used at the breakfast table.
- The cayenne pepper might seem unnecessary, but it is actually very important. Not only does it help to add a bit of a kick, but the pepper helps to break up mucus and increases healthy blood flow. It also is a good source of B and C vitamins, commonly

referred to as Super Vitamins due to their many benefits for the body.

- Mixing teas with the recipe is one way to help modify things, just make sure it's decaffeinated tea because caffeine can restrict blood vessels and we want to keep your body passages as open as possible.

These two drinks were the highlight of my day and I still use the Pineapple cocktail for breakfast. I now add bananas and a pinch of hot pepper, 2 pinches of turmeric powder, and 4-6 table spoons of hemp for protein.

A new research from Germany and the USA about a Pineapple cocktail. US Nutritionist Dr. Norman Walker till his age of 116 believed that his secret to a healthy long life is vitamins in liquid. His tip for free Radicals is: Pineapple for pure enzymes. It supports your immune system and kills cancer cells as well as tumors. The recipe: 3 rings of pineapple-fresh purred with one cup of cottage cheese 3 times per week.

Another favorite drink - grind 2 tablespoons of flax seeds (use a coffee grinder) or use 1 tablespoon of organic cold pressed flaxseed oil, ½ cup organic yogurt or ½ cup organic cottage cheese and 1 cup organic Concord grape juice. Blend and drink. It's a great breakfast drink!

- **Hot Castor Oil Packs** – highly anti-viral, anti-bacterial, anti-cancer prevention – Every Night for 30 minutes for one month. It has been used for over 100 years to reduce, dissolve, break up tumors and cysts. OLD FASHION HOT WATER BOTTLE WHICH WILL INCUBATE THE MOIST HEAT – THEN THE FABRIC ON SKIN AND BOTTLE ON TOP TO KEEP HEAT AND MOIST FOR AT LEAST 30 MINUTES - USE NATURAL FIBRE – HEAT IN OVEN (NO MICROWAVE)

- **Baking Soda** – Skin Cancer – make with water and paste and put it on the area over night – use Aluminum free baking soda **BOB'S RED MILL** brand , 1 – 2 teaspoons in water is a power alkalizer (1 – 2 times a day) ADD TO ALKALINE WATER

WILLINGNESS TO CHANGE –
I now choose calmly and objectively to see my old patterns and I am willing to changes. I am teachable. I can learn. I am willing to change. I choose to have fun doing this. I choose to react as though I have found a treasure when I discover something else to release. I see and feel myself changing moment by moment. Thoughts no longer have any power over me. I am the power in the world. I choose to be free. All is well in my world!
~ Louise L. Hay

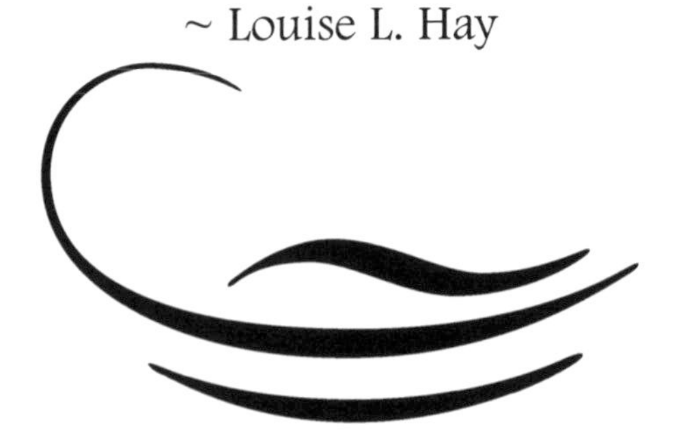

Chapter 15
The Need To Detox your Emotions!

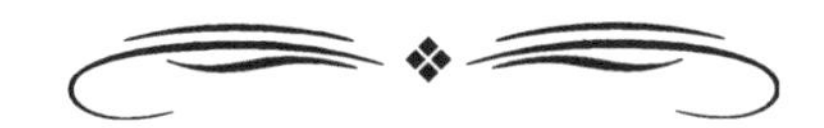

BY NOW, I HOPE YOU GET THE MESSAGE that everything you put into your body has an affect on your health. This goes for everything you put in your mind and your heart as well. We are all Body / Mind / Spirit interconnected. There's no getting around it. One affects the other, now, then, always and forever. So you have to detoxify your mind and emotions, too. This may be hard, and is usually done in groups because it's a little hard to bounce your issues off walls and get any viable feedback. It's possible, but it's much easier to do with another human being. I have listed all the organizations I could think of that would offer seminars on emotional cleansing, or emotional workshops. You'll have to contact them to see what's in your neighborhood. Research online. Research the counselors in your yellow pages.

Louise L. Hay – You Can Heal Your Life

Donna Eden – Energy Medicine

Masaru Emoto – The Hidden Messages In Water

I cannot stress enough how POSITIVE THINKING is INCREDIBLY important!

The truth may set you free,
but first it will shatter the
safe sweet way you live.
~ Ursula Kaiser

Chapter 16

Preventing the Cancer from Coming Back ~ STAYING CLEAN

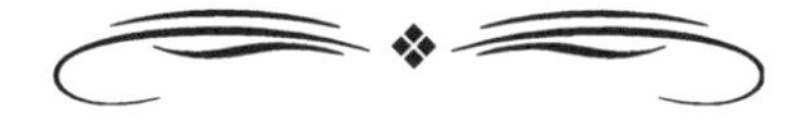

THIS SECTION IS ALSO FOR PEOPLE WHO have never had cancer. And want to make sure they never get it.

This is actually much easier and also much harder than it sounds. All you have to do is continue along this new lifestyle. Continue eating the correct acid/alkaline balance of foods, continue detoxing on a regular basis (I still do the coffee enema once per week), continue evaluating your feelings and recognizing when negative emotions are attacking. Sound like a lot? It is.

It's a new lifestyle. Welcome to the world of awareness. It's going to be up to YOU to be on top of your game every day. Nobody else is going to order the seaweed salad for you instead of the french fries.

It's helpful from time to time to see - in numbers - exactly how well we're doing. Sort of like a report card. The AMAS test from the ONCO lab is perfect for this. In the beginning do this test every 3 months. After one year of seeing your "passing" score, you can skip to every 6 months, and then to once per year. If ever your "score" is in the danger zone, go back to testing yourself every 3 months.

After a cancer diagnoses, take an AMAS test to see if you need more treatment. Or take it to monitor your progress after treatment.

Call 800-922-8378. AMAS can detect up to 18 months before any other test. This is FDA APPROVED; ask for a free kit to be sent to you. It detects cancer in an undiagnosed person up to 19 months before doctor's test can pick it up. In a cancer patient it allows a person to monitor the cancer activity in their body. Go to www.amascancer.com for additional information.

HOPE

In the darkest hour I found hope. Hope, to stop the tears from flowing. Hope to be here on earth for one more day. Please GOD that is all I am asking for. I promise to enjoy every moment.

~ Ursula Kaiser

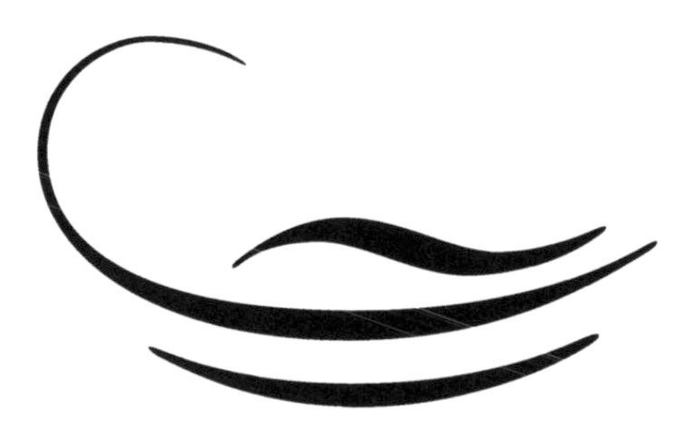

Chapter 17

Other Healing Modalities ...

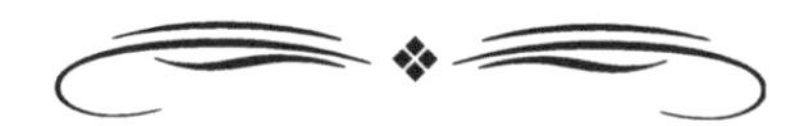

THE FOLLOWING IS A BRIEF PARAGRAPH about many, many different modalities and suggested therapies that are helpful in keeping body/mind/spirit cleansed and vibrant. Try all of them if you can. Choose as many as you can to do on a regular basis. Be creative. Incorporate them into your life. Many of these therapies can be done at home once you learn the basics.

Acupuncture is effective for immune stimulation and energy balancing.

Quantum Biofeedback SCIO Device or RIFE Energy Healing – Great tools to assist releasing negative energy from the body. Working with a local practitioner will allow you to evaluate, educate, and empower you to make the necessary lifestyle changes needed to reduce stress.

Research RIFE or Frequency Healing on the internet for further information. The full spectrum frequency machine uses specific frequencies to retune cellular signaling in order to restore optimal cell functions. Healthy cells and tissues radiate frequencies of a coherent nature. Diseased cells and tissues radiate frequencies of a chaotic nature. The Full Spectrum Frequency Machine is able to correct chaotic frequencies and turn them into a coherent integrated whole. When these corrections are made on an energetic level, the body can go about healing itself on a physical level. Normal cells are strengthened. The mutated cells are destroyed. Anything unnatural in the body causes an imbalance and is considered a foreign object by the immune system. This machine covers the entire spectrum of different frequencies so that all dysfunctional cells are addressed via a controlled delivery of specific frequencies.

The signal emitted by the Full Spectrum Frequency Machine is not steady nor constant, it is a controlled scan through a range of frequencies. There are two main settings the

Square Wave Mode and the Sine Wave Mode. Each setting emits waves for up to 20 feet, but it is recommended that you occupy the same room that the machine is in. You may cook dinner, watch TV, read, listen to the radio or visit with friends during treatment. Everyone benefits from this machine.

KNOWLEDGE IS POWER...

Healing Music – I used for my ovarian cancer "Flight of the Bumblebee." It can be found on the original Motion Picture Sound track Shine.

Soul & Spiritual Healing – It's very important to release all negative emotions and this means forgiving everyone that has hurt you as well as yourself for all of your past mistakes. What might you change in your life to enable you to heal?

Manual Lymphatic Massage - Manual Lymph Drainage is a very gentle type of massage therapy used to drain excess fluid from the body and improve the overall functioning of the lymphatic (immune) system. Most commonly used to treat Lymph edema, which is characterized by the blockage of lymph nodes in the arms and legs.

Energy Work – Reike – Body Talk – Quantum Biofeedback using SCIO, RIFE Frequency Machine, Scaler Wave

Yoga – Use Yoga as a way to reduce daily stress, enhance breathing, flexibility, and overall health and well being.

Chi Kung – Use Chi Kung will allow the body to restore itself. It oxygenates the body, enhances brain function, assists in moving blocked energy through the body, and reduces stress for overall health.

Pilates – Will assist in toning and tightening the body, enhances breathing, reduces stress, and improves overall health.

Meditation – Quieting the mind through meditation is a great place to start and will enhance balancing your overall chakra system for health and wellness.

Rest and Sleep

Sunlight

Beaches & Mother Nature – Walking barefoot and actually being grounded to mother earth is very healing.

Laughter – very important to laugh at yourself as well as funny movies.

Pursuit of Joy... Find your own happiness and make it happen your way!

I let go of everything that I no
longer need. My consciousness
is now cleansed and my concepts
are fresh, new, and vital.
~ Louise L. Hay

Chapter 18
Diet Adjustments

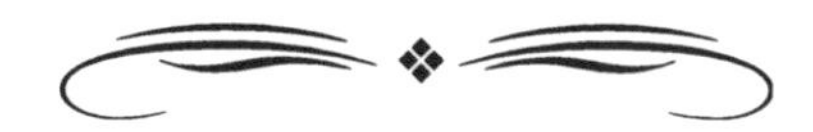

EXCESS SUGAR MUST BE ELIMINATED. Sugar feeds candida, cancer and chronic infections. Fruit juices feed candida. Proteins are OK. White flour and anything made from white flour should be eliminated. A good rule of thumb is DO NOT EAT anything white. Green is best for you. Try to stop ingesting all chemicals and preservatives as they contribute to liver toxicity and cause free radical damage. Eat natural whole foods, organic, if possible. Drink plenty of the best water possible. NO DIET SODAS. No Aspartame, No MSG. Work to make you body more alkaline.

Cancer loves an acidic body!

Eat a few organic fruits and lots of organic vegetables, often. Eat raw veggies if possible. Otherwise lightly steam them. If you have a juicer, consider juicing a variety of veggies. Green is the best for you! Suggestion for juicing any combination of parsley, broccoli, cauliflower, cabbage, kale, Swiss chard, cilantro and spinach. A few carrots, or apples sweetens this drink up and tastes very good to me.

I always add one lemon and a small piece of fresh ginger to my green drink.

FOODS TO RESTRICT IN YOUR DIET

1. All Processed Refined Foods **(Rule - if man made it DON'T EAT IT)**
2. Alcohol
3. Tobacco
4. All Conventionally Grown Meats, Vegetables & Fruits
5. Table Salt
6. Refined Sugar
7. All Sodas and Carbonated Beverages

8. Coffee & Black Tea
9. Dairy Products unless properly cultured (i.e. Kiefer or Organic Cottage Cheese)
10. All Pastries, Sweets, Candy, Ice Cream, etc.
11. Flour Based Products
12. Preserved Foods
13. Unfermented Soy

I am free; I release the past.
Life flows easily through me.
I release all pressure and
burdens. I live in the
joyous present.
~ Louise L. Hay

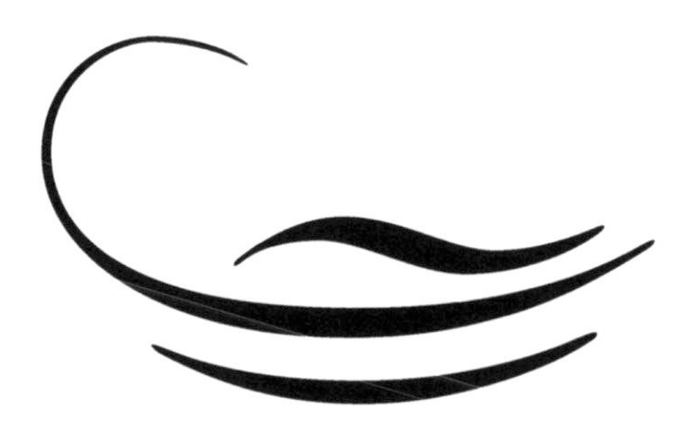

Chapter 19
Tips for Prevention

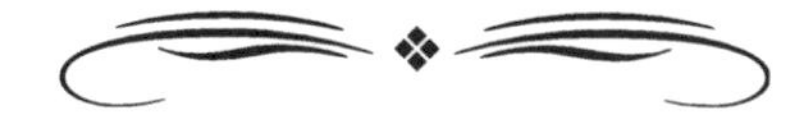

1. Having a Good Foundation is the best way to PREVENT Cancer

2. Wholesome Whole Food Daily Diet

3. 6 – 8 servings of vegetable and fruits a day

4. Veggie Juices

5. Smoothies

6. Maintenance Cleanses to keep the system pure – every 3 months – just like you change your oil every 3000 miles.

7. Think Natural NO CHEMICALS

8. Reducing Toxic Exposure – Assess Environmental Factors Where you Live – Industrial – Power Lines – etc.

9. Reduce Physical Stress

10. Eliminate Emotional Stress

11. Proper Hydration

12. Proper Rest

13. Tumeric Powder add to Juices

14. Exercise – Breathing – Yoga

15. Healthy Gums thru Oil Pulling – Traditional Virgin Raw Coconut Oil - Google Oil Pulling written by a Dentist

16. Sun Light – Vitamin D – Grounding (touch the actual earth which grounds our magnetic body.) The Beach is great source of negative ions.

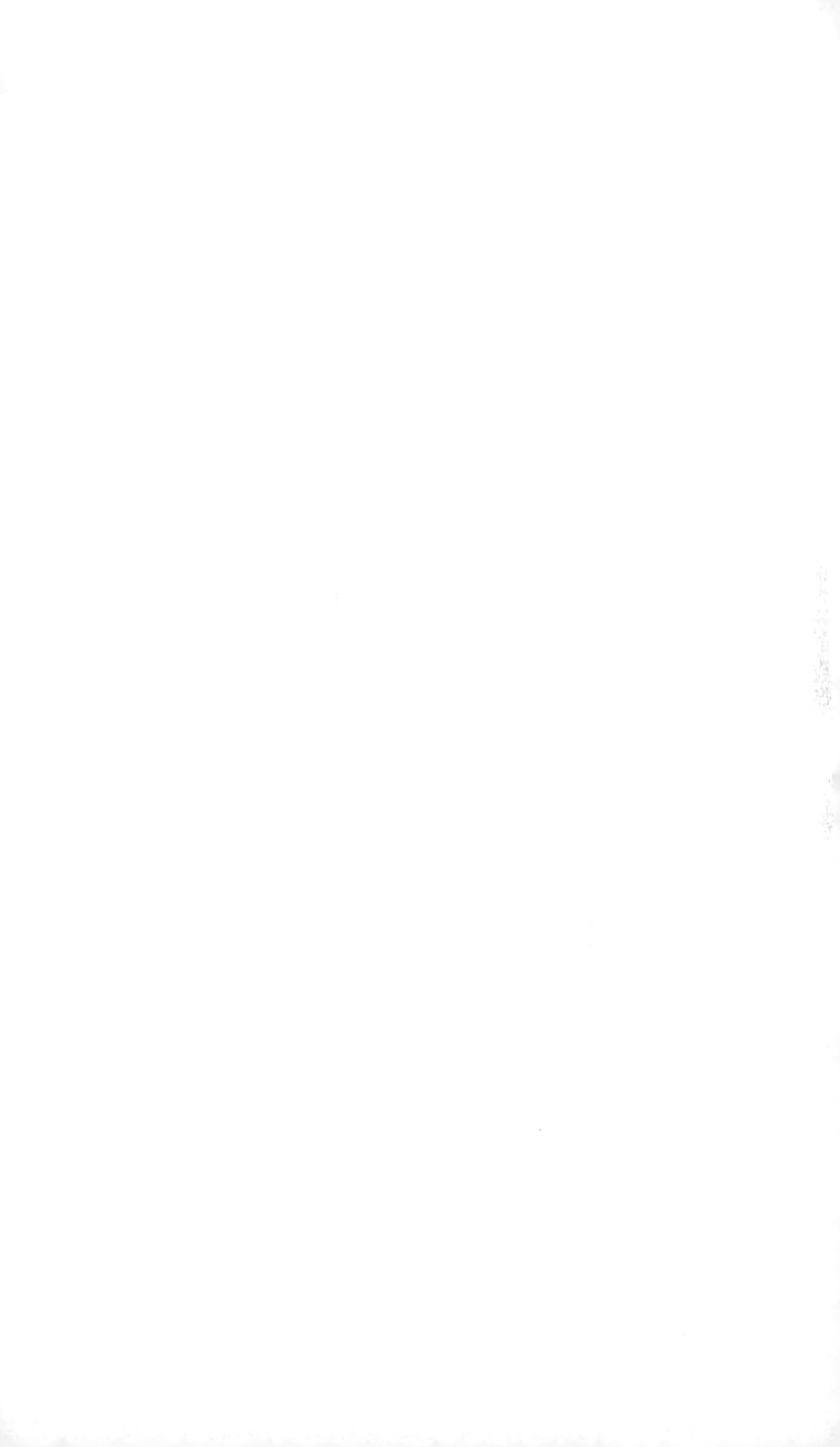

I accept health as the natural state
of my being. I now consciously release
any mental patterns within me that could
express as disease in any way. I love and
approve of myself. I love and approve of
my body. I feed it nourishing foods and
beverages. I exercise it in ways that are
fun. I recognize my body as a wondrous
and magnificent machine and I
feel privileged to live in it. I love lots of
energy. All is well in my world.
~ Louise L. Hay

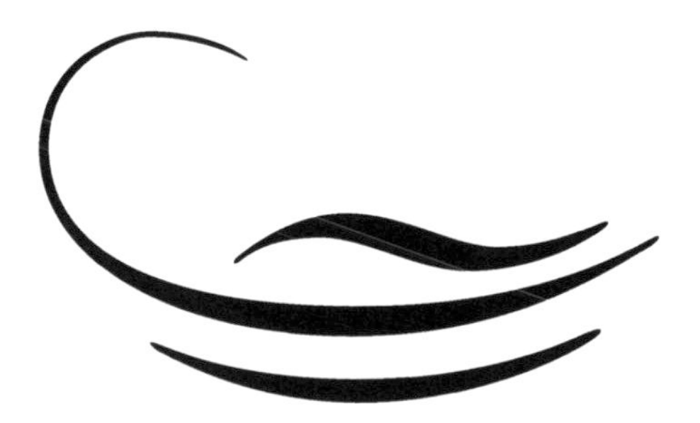

Chapter 20

Quick Start for Health & Wellness Naturally

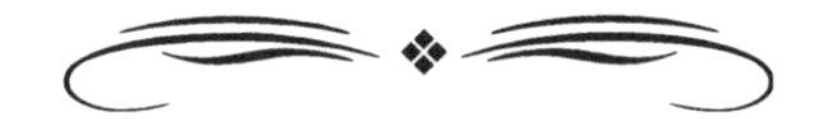

1. Do All Cleanses First

2. Essiac Tea Every Day

3. Baking Soda – Alkalines the Body Immediately

4. Baking Soda is great for Skin Cancer – make with water a paste and put it on the area overnight.

5. Castor Oil Packs - highly anti-viral, anti-bacterial, anti-cancer prevention – Every Night for 30 minutes for one month (see details in Cleanse section).

6. Hydration Drinking Enough Good Water – ½ body weight in ounces of fluid EXAMPLE 100 lbs. is 50 ounces of water to drink!

7. Baking Soda – Alkaline the Body Immediately – 2 x a day

8. Juicing Daily

9. Smoothies Daily

10. Coffee Enema Daily or Peroxide Enema (colon enema) up to 100 drops (only food grade 35%) Food & Thought Naples, FL $9.00 to purchase if you cannot find locally

11. Sweat Therapies – Sauna Hot Baths Work Out – Cleanses the Body

12. Move Negative Energy Out

13. Deep Breathing Exercises to release tension oxygenates the brain and body and so much more!

14. Meditation

15. Laughter

16. Pilates – Yoga – Chi Kung
17. German Drinks - Flaxseed Oil, organic concord Grape Juice, Cottage Cheese.
18. Essential Vitamins and Minerals thru Green Powder - Super Food – or whatever the best one you can find in your local store.
19. High Volume of Vitamin C – (increase dosage until the bowels loosen, then back off)
20. Lugo's Iodine by Southern Botanicals in Clearwater, FL Go to www.healthfree.com

Chapter 21
Reference Books To Read

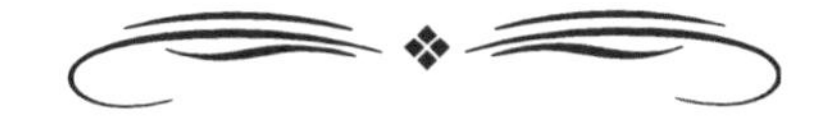

Louise L. Hay – "You Can Heal Your Life"

Donna Eden – "Energy Medicine"

Masaru Emoto – "The Hidden Messages In Water"

Bill Henderson – "CANCER-FREE"

Charlotte Gerson with Beata Bishop – "HEALING the Greson Way"

Patrick Quillin - "Beating Cancer with Nutrition"

David R. Hawkins – "Power vs. Force: The Hidden Determinants of Human Behavior"

Donald Kelly – "One Answer to Cancer"

Dr. Moss – "Antioxidants Against Cancer"

Dr. Moss – Antioxidants Against Cancer THE DOCTOR WHO CURES CANCER by William Kelley Eidem.
Published by Huge Health Secrets.
The story of Emanuel Revici, M.D.
The Mexican clinic is Hope 4 Cancer Institute, USA # 800 544-5993.
Dr. Tony Jimenez is the Medical Director.

Holistic Health Solutions located in Naples , Florida
For Clients for whom health is the top priority, consider contacting Holistic Health Solutions in Naples, FL. Richard Campanella has been helping clients achieve optimal health in his holistic health clinic for years and has helped many very ill people to take charge of their own health. He is available to assist you in setting up a healing center in the comfort of your own home. Please call 239.566.1210 or www.HolisticHealthSolutions.com for more information.

OTHER WEBSITES TO REVIEW

www.CancerDecisions.com

www.Mercola.com -
The Illegal Herb that Fights Cancer Article

www.CancerSuccessForum.com

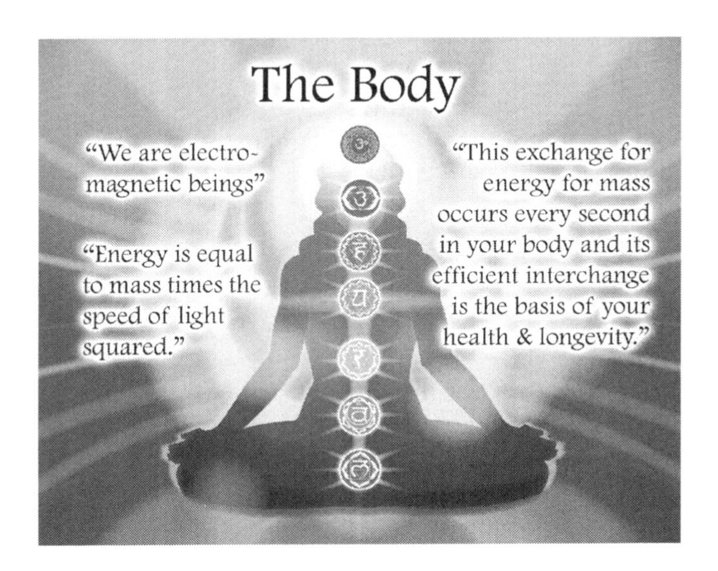

The light of God surronds us.
The love of God enfolds us.
The power of God protects us.
And the presence of God watches over us.
Wherever we are, GOD is.
And all is well.
~ Unity Prayer

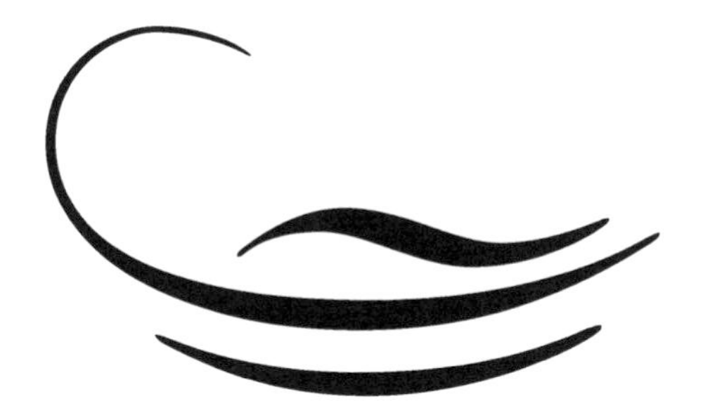

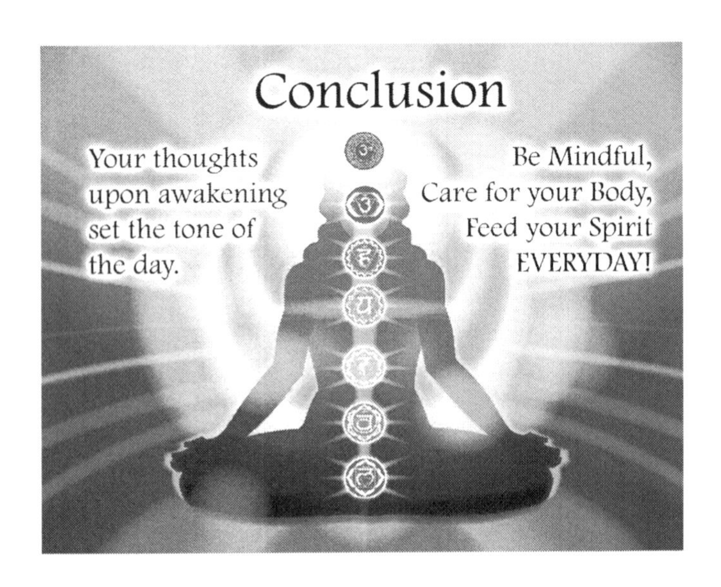

Loving everything about yourself even the unacceptable – it's an act of personal power. It is the beginning of healing.
~ Christane Northrup, MD

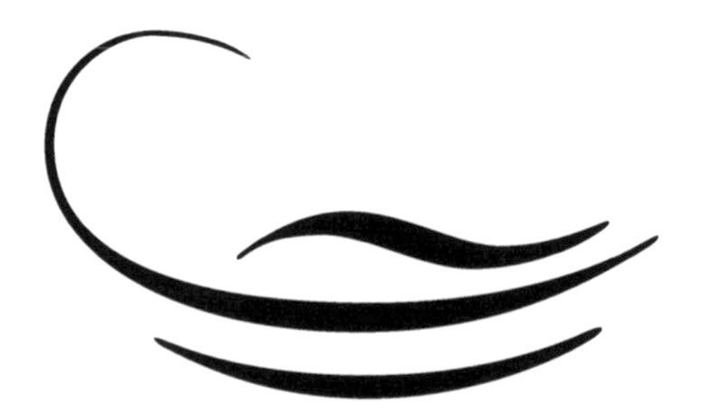

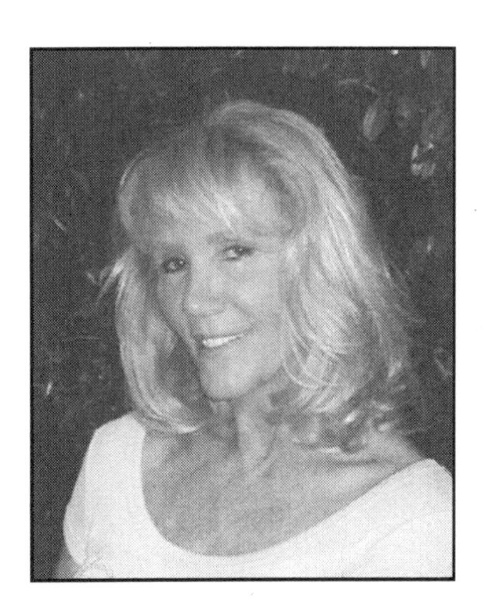

ABOUT THE AUTHOR

Ursula Kaiser was born in the small town of Rendsburg, Germany, near the Danish border. At age ten she organized an all-girl handball team (11 in the field in summer and 7 indoors, almost like basketball here in the States.) At a young age, she had Fernweh, "far away dreams," and when she left, she was never homesick.

Her dream was to travel the world and move to America, Australia, Canada, or South Africa. At age 19 and still in business school, she applied for jobs in those countries and was accepted in New York. That city was way too big, so she moved to a smaller city-town, Chicago, which was more manageable. Ursula worked three jobs, saved money, and bought a company that imported kitchen utensils from Europe.

Ursula met her husband in Chicago. They married in 1972 but she lost him five years later, to ill health. She was still highly motivated, and put all of her energies into her business and career. When the dollar weakened, she bought a small manufacturing company in Chicago that designed unique kitchen utensils.

Ursula has appeared on ***Good Morning America*** and several cooking shows. She designed and sold baking products to Martha Stewart. She worked with many department and gourmet stores in the US, and exported her products to Europe, Japan, and Australia. She traveled all over the globe for trade shows and loved the cooking industry. Cooking became her hobby, in addition to tennis, biking, roller blading, and skiing.

Life was great until a long, drawn-out business lawsuit and court battle took its toll on her health, wellness, and life. Ursula believes that, due to the high stress of this lawsuit, she attracted cancer to her body, even while living a healthy lifestyle.

Ursula then went on her journey to Health and Wellness, naturally. Her credentials are surviving a death sentence and doing her own due diligence. She has logged in thousands of hours of research to find natural ways of healing, using the techniques and technologies she shares in this book.

She hopes you will find some peace of mind in knowing you can heal yourself naturally, if that is your path. She hopes you use her resources and insights on how important it is to cleanse your entire mental, emotional, physical, and spiritual body to regain your life, and stay there, too!

Ursula is available to lecture and coach you to VICTORY over any health issue you may have. All you need to do is ask.

IN LOVE AND LIGHT...
TO YOUR HEALTH AND WELL BEING!

Dear Reader,

Thank You for allowing me to share my Journey To Wellness. I hope it has inspired and empowered you to follow your intuition to heal naturally. I send my love and healing energy your way and know that we are always connected.

I wish you health, happiness, and HOPE!

Made in the USA
Charleston, SC
23 August 2011